STRESS
& Health
SECOND EDITION

To my parents

STRESS
& Health
Biological and Psychological Interactions

SECOND EDITION

WILLIAM R. LOVALLO
University of Oklahoma

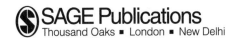
SAGE Publications
Thousand Oaks ▪ London ▪ New Delhi

5405000386698

12th SEPTEMBER 2012

For information:

Sage Publications, Inc.
2455 Teller Road
Thousand Oaks, California 91320
E-mail: order@sagepub.com

Sage Publications Ltd.
1 Oliver's Yard
55 City Road
London EC1Y 1SP
United Kingdom

Sage Publications India Pvt. Ltd.
B-42, Panchsheel Enclave
Post Box 4109
New Delhi 110 017 India

Printed in the United States of America

Library of Congress Cataloging-in-Publication data

Lovallo, William R.
Stress and health : biological and psychological interactions / William R. Lovallo.—2nd ed.
    p. cm.
Includes bibliographical references and index.
ISBN 13 978-1-4129-0478-0 (pbk.)
    1. Stress (Physiology) 2. Stress (Psychology) I. Lovallo, William R. Stress & health. II. Title.
QP82.2.S8L68 2005
616.9'8--dc22   2004013648

      08   09   10   9   8   7   6   5   4

Acquiring Editor:	Jim Brace-Thompson
Editorial Assistant:	Karen Ehrmann
Production Editor:	Sanford Robinson
Typesetter:	C&M Digitals (P) Ltd.
Copy Editor:	Elisabeth Magnus
Indexer:	Teri Greenberg
Cover Designer:	Ravi Balasuriya

Contents

Preface

This book is an introduction to the concept of psychological stress, its physiological manifestations, and its effects on health and disease.

When preparing the first edition, I told a former student that I was writing a book on stress. She replied, "What, *another* book on stress?" Indeed, the topic of stress is widely covered in the lay media and in academic writings, and a reader may well ask why we need another book on the subject. I sense that there are two reasons.

First, it is widely believed that stress is a significant factor in our lives and that it may contribute to illness. This view has a history going back at least as long as people have suffered, and it is a guiding principle in the field of health psychology. For this reason, it seemed timely and useful to make available a readable account of the specific linkages between emotions and physiological changes.

Second, in reviewing books and papers available to the student and the general professional audience, I noted a complete absence of any text dealing with the question of stress physiology and its integrations with thoughts and emotions. Instead, the material was often found only in highly specialized sources, and it appeared in fragmented form, scattered in review articles and chapters. This fragmentation places an undue burden on the reader to assemble a wide range of incompatible materials written at varying levels of detail, for various purposes, and with differing viewpoints. As a result, it becomes unnecessarily difficult for students and working professionals to develop an understanding of the pathways by which thoughts and emotions affect the body.

This book developed from a course I have taught at the University of Oklahoma Health Sciences Center on Stress and Disease. That course stemmed from my interest in helping graduate students in biological psychology understand how stress affects the body and how these processes may alter long-term health. Most important, I sensed the need to attend carefully to the biological links between how we think and feel and the changes in brain function that accompany these thoughts and feelings. As a result, this book concentrates on the psychophysiological linkages between cognitions, emotions, brain functions, and the peripheral mechanisms by which the body is regulated.

A second interest I had in my course was to enhance the integration of the stress concept into a larger framework by presenting its historical context and its relationship to the development of medicine. Although we have an increasingly clear understanding of the machinery of the body and its systemic dysregulation in disease, medicine in its traditional formulation lacks a conceptual approach to understanding how social processes and emotions can improve or worsen health. We therefore start and finish this book with a brief historical discussion of the mind-body relationship in terms of the development of our current system of medicine. I believe that exposure to these broader questions will provide students with a more complete awareness of the potential contributions that behavioral medicine can make to the study of health and disease.

The presentation here is intended for undergraduate and graduate students of psychology, physiology, behavioral medicine, anthropology, nursing, the neurosciences, and related fields who are interested in a broad introduction to these topics. There will also be selected areas where more advanced students and working professionals may discover new information or enjoy a useful review. I have assumed that most readers have a background in basic psychology and at least one course in basic biology, physiology, or physiological psychology. Chapters 4 through 9 assume an exposure to human neuroanatomy, neurophysiology, and some autonomic and endocrine physiology. For readers lacking such background preparation, I have avoided the use of specialized terms without explanation, and I have referred to background sources where it seemed appropriate.

This book should be useful in basic courses in health psychology for undergraduates and graduates alike. It may serve as a stand-alone text or as a basis for more extensive coverage of each topic, supplemented by appropriate readings.

In preparing this second edition, I was struck by the extent to which the first edition has continued to be a useful resource. It continues to serve teachers needing a brief text to anchor courses in behavioral medicine, and it has provided students in related fields a helpful introduction to a topic often available only through numerous specialized publications that can be intimidating to the newcomer or others wanting a consolidated source of information. I was also struck by the enduring usefulness of some of the basic formulations provided in the first edition.

Chapter 6 in the earlier edition combined neural and autonomic outflow mechanisms with stress endocrine regulation. In the 7 years since that chapter was written, the research on glucocorticoid regulation, its effects on the body and its feedback effects on the brain, has begun to accelerate. For this reason, the material on endocrine regulation has been expanded into an entire chapter, thereby providing room to indicate some of the new directions in which researchers have taken this field.

The other area where material has been expanded is in the rapidly emerging topic of stress interactions with gene expression. The past several years have witnessed an emergence of successful integration of the worlds of molecular biology and behavior. In response to this, I have provided a new chapter that deals with examples of this emerging paradigm. Fortunately for me, the material at hand was compelling enough to make a couple of stories that I enjoyed retelling and that I hope the reader will enjoy reading.

Knowledgeable readers will no doubt find one or more of these short chapters unsatisfactory because the material is covered too thinly or in too much detail or because the reader's favorite research is ignored or not referenced fully enough. Perhaps an editorial note is in order. When I was preparing the first edition, the excellent editor of the early volumes in this series, Rick Turner, and I made a couple of decisions that put a direction to the method of writing for this and other volumes in the series. We thought that the books should be brief and accessible to novices in their respective topics. This seemed to call for a modified textbook approach. We decided to present much research as factual knowledge with a minimum of referencing. This improved the flow of the exposition while avoiding the dry documentary style that burdens much academic writing. The intent was to provide sources with each chapter that would point the reader to more detailed and in-depth sources that were highlights in the literature.

This book is an introduction. It is not the last word or even the whole story; no single source, particularly one for students, could be. The result is that many topics are sparsely referenced or covered in an admittedly idiosyncratic manner. My shortcomings and omissions may at least provide many who use the book as a teaching aid opportunities to expand productively on its contents with assigned readings. For the self-taught reader, I hope the recommended readings will point you in the right directions and fill in these unavoidable gaps. Most important, I hope that all readers will gain enthusiasm for pursuing the topic further.

William R. Lovallo
Oklahoma City

Acknowledgments

Many of the ideas that have found expression in this second edition were first discussed by me and my colleagues at the University of Oklahoma in a long-running series of seminars on the neurobiology of stress held in the Behavioral Sciences Laboratories at the Veterans Affairs Medical Center. A great share of the credit for these seminars goes to my very good colleague Dean Myers, PhD, who was the co-leader of this series for 7 years. Similarly, I thank my colleague Beverley Greenwood, PhD, who contributed greatly to the content and quality of the seminars. Elliot Ross, MD, an accomplished neurologist with a passion for the central organization of the emotions, was an inspiration not only in helping me think through the topic of the emotions but also in improving my knowledge in neuroanatomy. The mistakes, of course, are all mine.

During the 1980s and 1990s, an outstanding group of graduate students passed through the Behavioral Sciences Laboratories. In addition to their enthusiastic involvement in our seminar series, these students provided intellectual challenge and stimulation on a daily basis. They should have some credit for the development of some of these ideas, at least the best parts. In particular, I mention Susan Everson, Andrea King, Mustafa al'Absi, Tony Buchanan, Robert Miranda, and Jack Shepard.

While writing the first edition, I had the privilege of serving as the associate director of the MacArthur Foundation's Research Network on Mind-Body Interactions. I thank my fellow network members for their personal examples and for their highly stimulating dialogue, which has continued to find its way into this volume in a number of places. I also thank Bob Rose, the network's director, for his generous support while I was doing the bulk of the initial writing.

I am especially grateful to those who commented on specific sections of the first edition of this book and encouraged me to continue in that effort, and who therefore must have thanks for the contents of this second edition, including Mustafa al'Absi, Stephan Bongard, Michael Giordano,

Tom Hall, Anne Harrington, John Sheridan, and Jay Weiss. I extend my most sincere gratitude to the first editor of this series, J. Rick Turner, who was a constant source of encouragement and a superb judge of style and substance. Similarly I am most indebted to my colleague and former student Sue Everson, who provided very constructive criticism, greatly enhancing the value of several chapters. I am similarly grateful to persons who read the book for their own interest or were assigned it for classes and who took the trouble to give constructive criticism and helpful suggestions for future editions.

Finally, I must thank the U.S. Department of Veterans Affairs, an organization often unheralded for its generosity to its researchers, for giving me a wonderful place to work for the past 31 years.

1

Behavioral Medicine
and Biomedicine

I n 1928, the American physiologist Walter Cannon was addressing the
Massachusetts Medical Society on the subject of emotions and disease.
He recounted:

> A wife who was free from any cardiac disorder saw her husband walking
> arm in arm with a strange woman and acting in such a way as to rouse jeal-
> ousy and suspicion. Profoundly stirred by the incident the wife hastened
> home and remained there several days. She then began to fear going out lest
> she might meet her husband with her rival. After days of wretchedness
> she was persuaded by a friend to venture forth, "probably in a state of abject
> terror," . . . but she had not gone far when she ran back to her home. Then she
> noted that her heart was thumping hard, that she had a sense of oppression
> in her chest and a choking sensation. Later attempts to go outdoors produced
> the same alarming symptoms. She began to feel that she might die on the
> street if she went out. There was no organic disease of the heart, and yet
> slight effort as she moved from her home brought on acute distress. (p. 881)

It is always impressive to see how the impact of a psychologically
meaningful event can change a person's physical state. Examples like this
lead us to ask, "How can an idea change the body?"

This book is concerned with mental activity and behavioral processes
and their relationship to states of health and disease. We specifically take
up the question of psychological stress and describe how mental activity
can produce negative effects on the body, perhaps leading to disease

or even death. We also present research indicating how the effects of psychological stress can be buffered by early experiences, leaving the individual better able to withstand stresses and strains of life. These positive examples are few, and they suggest that much more is known about vulnerability to stress than about hardiness or resilience.

We mentioned that this book was about mental and behavioral processes. When we say *behavior*, we mean not only moving and talking but also the neural processes giving rise to thoughts and emotions. Ideas about the relationship between the mind and the body have been debated since the ancient Greeks. In fact, the mind-body problem is one of the fundamental philosophical and scientific issues in human knowledge. Integrating our thinking about behavior and mental life into our thinking about medicine is essential to developing a truly behavioral medicine.

Although our example above is true to life and perfectly understandable as a reaction, we have little understanding of *how* this woman's seeing her husband with his girlfriend led to such extreme fear and to her physical symptoms. Since 1928, we have become increasingly familiar with the mechanisms of the brain and how these control the rest of the body. Similarly, psychology has increased our knowledge about how we learn, think, and take in the world. Still, studies of the workings of the body and the processes of the mind seem to exist in separate departments at our universities and in separate compartments of our thinking. This division keeps us from understanding our woman patient and the relationships between her experience, her emotions, and her physical state. In considering behavioral influences in health and disease, we need to have a way of thinking about how words can affect the body. We understand how bacteria and viruses can invade our bodies and how heart disease develops in the arteries of the heart, but we are not yet fully comfortable with the idea that psychological processes such as emotions and personality characteristics can influence these same disease processes.

This book is a short review of how our behaviors, especially ideas and associated emotions, come to have power over our bodies. It is an attempt to create a model of the psychological stress response in relation to its biological consequences. In the process, we hope to gain some useful insights into how psychological theory can contribute to our view of medicine.

To make sense of the concept of psychological stress and its place in behavioral medicine, we begin by briefly addressing the development of modern Western medicine. In Chapter 2, we sketch some newer approaches to an understanding of behavioral interactions with health and disease. Chapter 3 briefly reviews the history of the stress concept, and Chapter 4 discusses physiological regulation by way of the autonomic nervous system and the endocrine system. In Chapter 5, we make an important distinction between "physical" and "psychological" stress reactions that is frequently overlooked, with some resultant misunderstanding among researchers and laypersons. In Chapter 6, we move to an examination of the brain processes that instantiate the psychological stress response. The psychological-physiological distinction is developed further in a discussion of appraisal processes and how these may contribute to the patterning of brain activity seen in negative emotions and states of distress. Chapter 7 revisits the cortisol response that accompanies states of distress. This base of information is necessary for understanding how feedback from the body can permanently alter brain function, so it is part of a crucial discussion of why some stressors may be beneficial and some harmful. Chapters 6 and 7 thus form the core of this book. They lead naturally to a consideration of how people differ in their responses to stress. Chapter 8 presents a brief description of the immune system and presents research on the emerging discipline of psychoneuroimmunology, which studies how thoughts and feelings may be related to the risk for infectious and inflammatory disease. Chapter 9 discusses the concept of helplessness and evidence that loss of control has particularly devastating effects on the individual. Chapter 10 is entirely new. It deals with the now rapidly emerging topic of genes and behavior. With regard to stress and stress reactivity, there are now outstanding examples of how the development of individuals, animal or human, can be altered profoundly by their unique experience in light of their genetic endowment. Chapter 11 discusses the differences between persons in stress reactions, how these differences may relate to brain function, and how experience may shape these differences. It is hoped that a systematic top-down look at the brain and organization of the stress outputs to the body via the autonomic and endocrine systems will provide an organized way of thinking about reactivity. Chapter 12 concludes this admittedly brief discussion on stress with considerations for the state of behavioral medicine and our understanding of how experience can have both positive and negative impacts on our health.

The Age of Enlightenment and the Emergence of Scientific Thought

Our task is to understand the role of the brain in health and disease. Modern medicine—what we might call biomedicine—represents one of the major successes of science. Our science is a product of our Western worldview. We will therefore examine this worldview and the kind of science that emerged from it. In the process, we may see how it is difficult for traditional Western biomedicine to provide for the treatment of patients like the woman in our example.

The current worldview can be considered to date from the 17th century, at the end of the Renaissance and the beginning of the Age of Enlightenment. However, we didn't suddenly invent our world in the 1600s, so we begin by addressing ideas developed before that time and how they continue to shape our worldview today. At present, we think of ourselves as modern persons who must surely see things differently than the Greeks did, but in fact we often embellish ancient concepts without replacing them.

The Greeks saw reality as having two fundamentally different aspects: One was the physical world, perceived through our senses. The other was the world of ideas, the intelligible world of true knowledge. Reachable through reason alone, this unchangeable world of pure forms was thought to form the ideal essence of the physical world. The philosopher, according to Plato (1964), pursued "the knowledge that reveals eternal reality, the realm unaffected by change and decay" (p. 274). The visible world, in contrast, was changeable and illusory. Much of Western thought has retained this deeply rooted belief that the world consists of an illusory surface and an underlying nonphysical perfection.

For Plato, there were four ordered classes of reality. First, there were shadows and reflections of things in the world as perceived through our senses. These were seen as subject to illusion and misinterpretation. Second came true objects, somewhat more certain but still subject to the vagaries of our fallible senses. Third came the sciences, which were more certain in their foundation than sensory experience but still subject to revision and refinement. Fourth, there was the world of pure ideas, the world of true essences of physical objects (Plato, 1964).

Two important themes emerge from this brief description of Greek thought. First, the Greeks placed great value on the power of human reason to understand nature—an idea that we also hold. Second, the Greeks had a metaphysically dualistic view of the world. Everything had its essential qualities and its physical qualities. The world of the mind was not the physical world.

The Renaissance (approx. 1300 to 1600), the period that emerged from the Dark Ages (approx. 450 to 1100), was marked by the rediscovery of ancient learning and the reemergence of classical Greek thought. During the Enlightenment, which represented the emergence of reason over belief, we can see clearly the traces of this metaphysical dualism. At the beginning of the 17th century, the rational study of nature was becoming an important means to gain knowledge, but as science emerged it came into conflict with the older, prevailing religious sentiment, which dictated that true knowledge was handed down and not discovered through reason alone. René Descartes (1596–1650), the 17th-century French philosopher and mathematician, made historic contributions to epistemology and mathematics, and by the time of his death we could say that all of the main pieces of our modern worldview were in place. He provided the philosophical beginnings of modern science and medicine, but he left the Greek dualism in place in order to deal with the religious and political realities of his time.

Descartes and the Mechanical Model of Living Things

Descartes established the core principles of modern scientific epistemology, nicely summarized in his book *Discourse on Method* (1637/1956). Epistemology answers the question "How do we know that our knowledge is valid?" The adoption of a particular epistemology determines how we might go about acquiring knowledge, what sorts of theories about the world are legitimate.

In the *Discourse*, Descartes addressed the question of how to study the natural world. He strongly rejected any reliance on external authority as a source of received knowledge. For him, knowledge was valid only if based on careful observation informed by the use of reason. Most famously, he emphasized that the world could be seen as a series of objects interacting as a complex machine, much as a clock could be seen as a series of interacting springs, wheels, gears, and levers. Also like a clock, the world could be disassembled into simpler subunits so that the machine's subassemblies could be studied. This reductionist approach to the study of natural phenomena is a hallmark of how science acquires new information. Its other essential characteristic is the reliance on experimentation and empirical observation to verify hypotheses and predictions, as forcefully espoused by Francis Bacon (1561–1626).

The problem for Descartes in establishing his epistemology was to address apparent differences between living things and inert matter, and between humans and other living things. Living things are spontaneous and, well, *alive*. Machines, on the other hand, just sit there and don't really do anything on their own. In addition, as living humans, we are aware of our thoughts and sensations, things surely denied to machines, even our modern computers. Most important, the body is made of physical matter, which eventually dies and disappears, whereas the soul was seen by Descartes and most contemporaries as nonphysical and immortal. This Greek-based view of human nature, inherited by

Descartes, is reinforced by our subjective sense of ourselves as having a nonphysical mind inhabiting our physical bodies (Ryle, 1949). Finally, Descartes had to confront the dominant power of his day, the Catholic Church, which held strongly to the Greek view of things and was prepared to severely punish anyone who taught a different view. For perhaps all of these reasons, Descartes (1637/1956) wrote, "I then described the rational soul, and showed that it could not possibly be derived from the powers of matter . . . but must have been specially created" (p. 38). We must note that what Descartes meant by the soul is very close to our view of the mind. In balancing his rational science with the prevailing belief system, Descartes managed to patch together a view of humans as biological machines inhabited by a nonmechanical soul that caused the machinery to move by acting through the pineal gland and then via microscopic tubes running through the nervous system to the muscles and internal organs.

Descartes moved science ahead by establishing the idea that we could take a mechanistic view of living things, but he left us with a significant conceptual problem by reserving a special place for our minds, arguing that they were subject to different laws than our bodies. This mind-body dualism has hindered our unified understanding of the relationship between what we call our psychological or mental existence and our physical presence. The split view of ourselves that we inherit from Descartes is the source of our difficulty in understanding how ideas can influence the body or how the mind can be an agent in health and disease.

We need to explore a little further how this Cartesian view of things influences our view of disease. We will start by thinking about the science that developed from Descartes's epistemology.

The Worldview and Premises of Modern Science

When we talk about our view of the fundamental nature of reality, we are talking about metaphysics. Western metaphysics, based on Descartes, goes something like this.

First, there is a single, fundamental, material level of reality. All things are made of increasingly complex assemblages of ordinary matter. Thus, it follows that more complex levels of organization do not involve *ontologically,* or fundamentally, new entities beyond the more basic elements of which they are composed. Put another way, more complex machines are simply combinations of simpler machines. They never become something fundamentally different from machines, no matter how subtle and complex they are. It also follows that there is a unified, *physicalist* language in whose vocabulary all phenomena subject to scientific inquiry can in principle be described. That is, we do not need a different language or set of scientific concepts to describe increasingly complex machines, even when these are biological organisms.

The second metaphysical principle deriving from the Cartesian mechanical view is that the material world has an external permanency over which nonmaterial activities (e.g., mental or physical activities) can have no effect. To make this point, Descartes (1937/1956) explicitly denounced claims of those who said they could move through time and space or levitate objects as the falsehoods of charlatans and magicians.

On the basis of these metaphysical principles inherited from Descartes and the early natural philosophers, science views the world in several specific ways. We can understand complex things by first studying their simpler parts (reductionism). The rules for such a study are derived from the same rules that explain mechanical objects (mechanism). Everything we observe has a physical cause (causality). Everything is therefore determined by some complex of causes (determinism). Last, we have inherited the unfortunate model of ourselves as beings with two natures, physical and spiritual (dualism). These points are discussed at length by Foss and Rothenberg (1988).

The Mind-Body Problem

Philosophers have noted the severe problems that arise when we hold to Descartes's dualism. Gilbert Ryle (1949) put it best:

> There is a doctrine about the nature and place of minds . . . prevalent among theorists and even among laymen.
>
> The official doctrine, which hails chiefly from Descartes, is something like this. . . . [E]very human being has both a body and a mind. Some would prefer to say that every human being is both a body and a mind. His body and his mind are ordinarily harnessed together, but after the death of the body his mind may continue to exist and function.
>
> Human bodies are in space and are subject to the mechanical laws which govern all other bodies in space.
>
> But minds are not in space, nor are their operations subject to mechanical laws.
>
> Such an outline is the official theory. I shall often speak of it, with deliberate abusiveness, as "the dogma of the Ghost in the Machine." (pp. 11–16)

This powerful dualistic position that Ryle ridiculed placed the emerging science of medicine in a physical framework from which the mind was largely excluded, and, in the mainstream of medicine, diseases were seen only in physical (and nonmental) terms.

Powerful as Descartes's mechanistic approach was to the study of living things, a minority of his contemporaries suspected that something was basically wrong with his mind-body dualism. Descartes had made the basic mistake of seeing matter as inanimate, unmoving, and incapable of behaving on its own without being moved by some outside force (Toulmin, 1967). Indeed, the inherent inertia of matter was the dominant view in Descartes's time, in line with Newton's mechanical model.

The minority view was best stated by Mettrie (1709–1751), who claimed that matter in reality was not dead, unmoving stuff. Mettrie saw matter as alive and argued that thought itself was not incompatible with the nature of matter (Toulmin, 1967). Descartes's mistake was in not recognizing that a fundamental property of matter was its ability to interact with itself and the world, to *behave*, if you will. An important conclusion from Mettrie's position was that living things did not need to be inhabited by some separate, mysterious mind-stuff to be able to think and act spontaneously. Instead, thinking and acting were behavioral properties that stemmed from the physical makeup of living things. Mettrie's position was and still is a radical view, and it was not widely shared at the time; it contrasted too sharply with the commonsense belief that physical matter was inert.

Claude Bernard and the Modern Biomedical Model

In spite of Descartes's strong views on the mechanical basis for the workings of the body, advances first occurred mainly in the physical sciences. Biology was left aside while physics and chemistry made rapid and important strides. Even by the mid-1800s, some believed that the workings of the body were impossible to study because of the invisible "vital forces" that occupied all living things. Claude Bernard (1813–1878) and other founders of modern physiology argued forcefully against this *vitalist* viewpoint (Bernard, 1865/1961). In line with Mettrie, Bernard insisted that living things obeyed all the same laws as nonliving things. Even though living things appeared to be self-moving and self-guided, this did not mean that they were inhabited by a nonphysical life force. For Bernard, the job of science was to learn to apply the laws of physics and chemistry to the new science of physiology.

Bernard's great contribution to medicine was to extend Cartesian epistemology and fully legitimize the study of living things as physical entities. However, the mechanistic model he promoted did not dispense with the dualism established by Descartes 200 years earlier. Though the mysterious life forces were done away with in the organs and muscles, they remained present in the brain in the form of our mental processes. This left us with a system of medicine based on physical principles, but from which the mind was excluded. With minor exceptions, this is the dominant view in our Western biomedical model. Although our viewpoint is gradually changing because of advances in the neurosciences and related biological and behavioral fields, this newer viewpoint is only beginning to gain ground in scientific medicine.

Our science of medicine has a physical basis. Disease is a physical condition. It exists apart from the observer, so the social organization or thoughts of the sick person have no effect on it. This view of disease as a physical process and our continuing belief that we have a nonphysical mind inside a machinelike body have made it difficult to develop a behavioral medicine. In a truly *behavioral* medicine, behavior, including our thoughts, feelings, and lifestyle, occupies the same conceptual space as our physical bodies. The mind-brain and the body influence each other, and our health and our behavior are part of the same process of life.

Summary

As the early scientists ruled out the existence of hidden forces in mechanical bodies in order to understand those bodies' functioning, so the pioneer physiologists banished vital forces from the body in order to understand its physical workings. However, just as Descartes made an exception in his epistemology for the claimed unique nature of the soul, Bernard and the later physiologists made an exception for the role of the mind in influencing the body. The mind, therefore, remained a mysterious, nonphysical presence inside our biological machinery.

The discussion of stress in later chapters will help clarify the nature of the relationship between the mind and the body. Recent advances in biology and the neurosciences give us a clearer picture of the inherently interactive—we may say behavioral—character of neurons and neuronal systems. This understanding gives us a basis for rethinking the relationship between the physical side of our nature and our mental existence.

Further Reading

Toulmin, S. (1967). Neuroscience and human understanding. In G. C. Quarton, T. Melnechuk, & F. O. Schmitt (Eds.), *The neurosciences: A study program* (pp. 822–832). New York: Rockefeller University Press.

A rich, powerfully informative, and concise discussion of the relationship between the study of the brain and the emerging reconceptualization of consciousness. These topics are fundamental to our understanding of how the mind can influence the body.

Bernard, C. (1961). *An introduction to the study of experimental medicine* (H. C. Greene, Trans.). New York: Collier. (Original work published 1865)

Bernard's writings are at once historically significant and highly entertaining as an account of the emergence of modern physiology. His work is the basis for our contemporary understanding of the workings of the body at rest and during stress.

Wozniak, R. H. (1992). *Mind and body: René Descartes to William James.* Bethesda, MD: National Library of Medicine.

Our discussion of the mind-body problem is very selective. Wozniak provides a thorough historical commentary on the major lines of thought related to this paradox during the development of modern psychology.

Fee, E., Sternberg, E. M., Harrington, A., & Brown, T. (1997). *Emotions and disease: An exhibition at the National Library of Medicine.* Bethesda, MD: Friends of the National Library of Medicine.

A well-written, concise, and illustrative catalogue of an exhibit at the National Library of Medicine that documents the historical shifts in our view of the mind and the body in medicine.

2

Psychosocial Models
of Health and Disease

W e know, or at least most of us believe, that we can't use our minds
   directly to influence outside objects. We can't levitate things. We
can't transport ourselves to another place by means of thought. Yet the
example at the beginning of the book reminds us that the mind influences
the body, sometimes in dramatic ways. How can we affect the state of
our body by our state of mind? That is the central question of this book.
In later chapters, we will concentrate on how the mind can create the
conditions for bodily stress responses, both acute and chronic. But before
we discuss specific psychological contributions to stress responses, we
should give thought to a more general conceptual model of how mental
processes can interact with processes of health and disease. This brief
consideration will allow us to place the topic of psychological stress in a
behavioral medicine framework. In addition, it will help us appreciate
how the behavioral medicine approach may complement and enrich a
more traditional medical model.

   We will start by analyzing the infectious disease process using a very
restricted biomedical model. We will show how this model can be usefully
expanded to include the behaviors of the patient. Then we will illustrate how
a behavioral medicine can be useful for understanding how placebo effects
operate. Finally, we will consider how a behavioral medicine approach
is especially helpful in conceptualizing cause and treatment in complex
diseases such as coronary artery disease.

The key concepts in this chapter are:

1. Disease processes should be seen as *dynamic interactions* between the causative agent and the affected organism.

2. The disease and its treatment are embedded in a *hierarchy* of systemic controls. That is, lower levels of the system are in two-way interaction with higher levels in the system, and each level integrates and regulates the levels below it. This point will be discussed in more detail in Chapter 4 as we describe the autonomic nervous system and higher controls in the brainstem and hypothalamus.

3. The hierarchy of causal influences ultimately includes *complex behaviors* such as the thoughts and emotions of the affected person and the socioculturally determined environment in which that person lives.

The Standard Biomedical Model and New Approaches to Medicine

In line with the Cartesian view, the standard biomedical model goes like this: Disease is a linearly causal process, "a condition of the living animal . . . or of one of its parts that impairs the performance of a vital function" (*Webster's Ninth New Collegiate Dictionary*, 1988). In other words, disease is disorder in an otherwise smoothly running machine. The cure is to disrupt the causative agent at the physical level to help the machine repair itself, restore order, and regain normal function. Finally, in the strong form of this model, following our Western tradition, the workings of the mind are irrelevant to the disease or its cure.

Figure 2.1 is a conceptual diagram of this strong form of the biomedical model. The diagram illustrates a normally functioning person being acted on by some pathogenic stimulus such as an infection, a cancer, or coronary heart disease. The mode of therapy is a direct physical intervention to restore the person's healthy, well-ordered state. Such therapy may be an antibiotic for a bacterial infection, chemotherapy for a cancer, or coronary bypass grafts for coronary heart disease. All of these treatments have known restorative, if not curative, properties. Their application in individual cases results in one of the three outcomes on the right. We hope that the patient gets better. However, other outcomes also occur, including continued illness or even death.

A key feature of this model is that the cure works with or without the knowledge or assistance of the patient. The cure is purely physical and

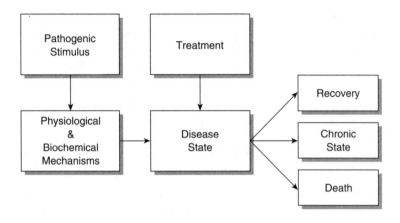

Figure 2.1   A restricted traditional medical model of the disease process. The disease process and the treatment are shown acting on a passive organism, and the treatment and disease do not interact.

not affected by the thoughts or emotional state of the person being treated. This traditional model has the following characteristics:

1. The model has *one-way causation.* The pathogen acts on the host and not the other way around.

2. The disease is a *physiological process,* and treatment operates on the physiology of the person to alter the disease state.

3. Therefore, the model is *nonhierarchical,* meaning that different levels of complexity in the system, particularly higher nervous system controls related to thoughts and emotions, do not interact with one another.

4. As a result, the model is *dualistic.* The mental status of the person is incidental to the cause of the disease and its cure. The mind and the body exist in different realms in this framework, and there is no strong basis for considering how they might work together for the person's well-being.

In considering the contrasting features of the biomedical model and the behavioral medicine model presented here, the following points should be kept in mind:

1. The traditional biomedical model has proven to be very effective at treating disease. When we speak of the shortcomings of the model, we mean that it is limited because it has no way to incorporate the knowledge that thoughts and emotions can enhance development of diseases or promote their cures.

2. Although those of us who consider emotions to be important in the health equation talk about the power of thoughts, these rarely, if ever, are the sole cause of disease. Instead, we think that such mental processes can alter the body in ways that may aggravate, or alleviate, otherwise existing disease processes.

3. We are only just beginning to understand how interactions between psychological processes and disease pathophysiology may occur. The information in this chapter is primarily a formal description of how such interactions may occur. Later chapters will deal with these interactions in more mechanistic fashion.

4. The study of behavioral influences on disease and its mechanisms must be approached with the same degree of scientific caution that is used in understanding disease and cure within the standard biomedical model.

This description of the traditional biomedical model and ways that it can be expanded is deliberately stark, allowing us to sharpen the contrast between approaches and to illustrate the potential contributions of a behavioral medicine. As individuals, doctors understand that the mind affects the body. They are well aware of the power of thoughts and emotions to affect health and the extent to which worry, grief, and anxiety can be obstacles to effective treatment. The problem for the physician is that the standard model by its nature does not provide a path for putting this intuitive knowledge into practice or for turning these mind-body relationships to the patient's advantage. Knowing that the mental state of the patient may affect the disease and response to treatment therefore becomes part of the art, rather than the science, of medicine, even in the hands of an insightful and empathetic practitioner.

Important areas of medical practice, such as family medicine, have a strong commitment to a *biopsychosocial model* of health. That is, they recognize the importance of the doctor-patient relationship, and treatment acknowledges that physical health is affected by psychological processes and by social conditions. Here, the physician has a philosophical commitment to appreciating the impact of social and psychological causes in health and disease and to bringing this understanding into the clinic. Unfortunately, little in standard medical training provides skills and knowledge in applying a biopsychosocial model.

The other side of this problem is that the emerging science of behavioral medicine is a promise not yet fully realized. There is a great deal of work to be done. Disciplines like psychology need to contribute to a base of theory and rigorously acquired knowledge that can lead to practical applications. This book will not solve the problem, but it will attempt to lay out what we know about the impact of psychological stress on the body, using an approach grounded in the neurosciences.

A Biobehavioral Model of Disease and Treatment

The model of disease outlined above is narrow. It restricts our view of the range of processes acting on our bodies, and this limits our thinking about the causes and therapeutic interventions possible in a behavioral medicine. We can expand our view of the disease process by embedding our first model in one that includes the person's learning history and sociocultural environment, as shown in Figure 2.2.

This expanded model of disease and treatment shows three important interactions between the person and the environment. First, the pathogenic stimulus interacts with the person's physiological and biochemical mechanisms. Not only does the pathogen affect the person's physiology, as in the traditional model, but the physiological and biochemical mechanisms of the host's immune system alter the pathogen. This interaction is primarily an *exchange of information* between host and pathogen.

According to current immunological knowledge about pathogen-host interactions, the pathogen provides information about itself to the host. This signals the immune system that a foreign organism is present and that the organism has certain proteins on its outer membrane, and it tells the immune system how to recognize these proteins. The immune system then seeks the foreign cells and attacks them with one or more defenses. In turn, the invader may have evolved counterdefenses to evade or trick the immune cells, allowing it to survive longer in the host.

The pathogen–immune system interaction illustrates how a wide range of behaviors, in this case at the cellular level, may play a role in the processes of disease and treatment. The host is involved in a *dynamic, interactive relationship* with the pathogen; this interaction is characterized by the *exchange of information* about the nature of the invader and the form of the host's defensive response; and the virulence of the infection is the outcome of the *interaction between the host and the pathogen.*

These interactions, exchanges of information, and virulence of the disease are *behavioral* interchanges. We normally think of behaviors as the overt actions of others and ourselves; we noted earlier that the term *behavior* should also include our inner thoughts and feelings. The idea that cellular interactions also have the characteristics of behaviors should not be disturbing because *behavior* is a good description of the interactive sequence of invasion, identification, cellular attack, and counterattack

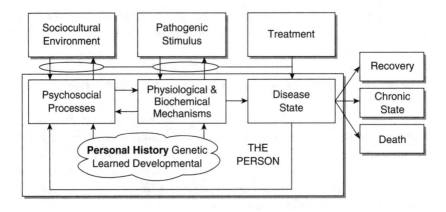

Figure 2.2   An expanded model of the disease process. The disease process interacts with the person, and psychological processes are shown interacting with physiological processes. In turn, the person interacts with the sociocultural environment. The treatment, disease, and environment can all interact as well.

involved in the infectious disease process. This expanded use of the term *behavior* readily allows us to incorporate the basic disease mechanism into a larger model including psychosocial and sociocultural processes, as we do in Figure 2.2. As we will see in Chapter 8, the dynamic properties of immune system behavior also provide abundant pathways for the study of interactions with higher nervous processes, such as emotions. For this reason, we have emphasized at several points the importance of seeing the disease and treatment as events in a hierarchically integrated system of behaviors and not as events isolated at the cellular or organ level.

Second, the person's psychosocial processes—his or her thoughts, emotions, and spoken words—interact with the sociocultural environment. Such *informational interchanges*—for example, concerning the nature of the disease and its cure—can affect treatment outcome.

It is not hard to imagine that the outcome of a pathogen's invasion will be different for a person whose learning history includes the knowledge of antibiotics, or whose preferred treatment calls for praying but not for visiting a physician. Knowledge of disease and choices of treatment are fundamentally informational and behavioral processes, just as the interactions between host and invader are informational and behavioral interactions at the cellular level. These learned and culturally conditioned information exchanges and behaviors determine the course and outcome of the disease just as the interactions at the immune system level do.

Finally, the treatment acts on the disease state, as in the traditional model. But the expanded model also incorporates the other person-environment interactions as processes that affect treatment outcome.

As Figure 2.2 shows, an important feature of the expanded model is that it is not linearly causal but recursive and interactive. In Figure 2.1, the arrows all point in one direction, suggesting that causation works in only one direction. In Figure 2.2, the two-way arrows invite us to think about the course of the disease and its treatment as repeated, or recursive, inter-actions. Disease and treatment become behavioral processes unfolding over time as an ongoing interchange between host and pathogen.

This model implies that treatment of an infectious disorder can have significant psychological, behavioral, and cultural elements. Note also the two-way arrows between psychosocial processes and physiological mechanisms, indicating that thoughts and emotions are intimately con-nected to the workings of our body; a clearer discussion of the mecha-nisms involved will be provided in Chapters 5 through 10. In a model such as this, *somatic disease, psychosomatic disease,* and *psychological disease* are no longer categorically different terms. They merely call our attention to different facets of the same process. From this perspective, the dualis-tic division of mind and body begins to break down. Some examples should indicate how our view of treatment, and even prevention, can change when we take such an expanded view of disease.

Placebo Effects

When a patient takes a preparation that has no known biological activity, yet the patient responds and perhaps improves, the preparation is called a placebo, from the Latin word meaning "I shall please," and the response is called a placebo effect. This implies that the medical effect has to do with a mental process associated with thoughts and emotions. In fact, the patient has to think that he or she is taking medicine to cure a specific disease. To understand placebo effects, we have to examine the informa-tion processes, including the beliefs and cultural norms of both the patient and the physician. When we consider the dynamics of placebo effects, we realize that all the interactions outlined in Figure 2.2 may accompany any form of treatment. That is, every form of treatment, placebo or other-wise, can have elements of psychological causation at work. This topic is discussed at length in engaging works by Benson and McCallie (1979),

Kirsch (1990), and Harrington (1997). The placebo effect illustrates the difficulties inherent in our tradition of mind-body dualism, and the controversy over how it works illustrates the difficulties of the biomedical approach in coming to terms with processes that start out in the psychological realm and end up in the body.

Current thinking is that placebos operate either because of the *expectancies* of the person receiving them or because of *conditioned associations* that may accompany the treatment situation. In both models, the initiating event is acknowledged to be psychological. Expectancies and conditioned associations, in turn, develop in a certain sociocultural environment and in persons with a certain learning history. We learn to expect things about the world from our culture and from our own experience. We have learned responses to the world we live in. A patient who is taking pills in a drug study but is unknowingly assigned to the placebo control group may think, "Doctors give people medicines that make them well. The pills I'm taking are designed to cure my illness. I have taken pills in the past that cured me of other illnesses, and perhaps these will work as well." These words describe expectations about what the pills might be able to do. In some cases, the ideas result in outright cures or therapeutic effects as large as those caused by the active drug, as discussed by Benson and McCallie (1979). For example, in various studies of medications for coronary heart disease, 33% to 37% of patients given placebos improved subjectively and objectively for up to a year or more—impressive results for an inactive compound.

This kind of outcome does not fit a traditional physicalist model of medicine. Placebo effects can be understood only as being mediated informationally by way of the central nervous system. Figure 2.3 illustrates that the traditional model of disease does not include a mechanism that permits physiologically inactive substances to have a measurable effect on the patient. There is no direct means by which the substance can intervene in the disease process.

This is not to say that traditional medicine ignores placebos, only that it has no metaphysical and epistemological bases for understanding them. The recognition that something occurs but that we have no means for conceptualizing or controlling it is uncomfortable, and it illustrates in another way the problem we have inherited with our dualistic metaphysics. An expanded model, such as the one in Figure 2.2, is more inclusive and opens up possibilities for incorporating placebo effects into our thinking. We can now begin to consider how experience, beliefs, and cultural norms might set the stage for physical changes to occur following ingestion of an otherwise inert substance in a treatment context.

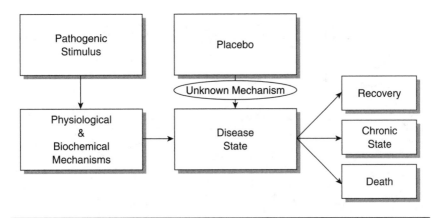

Figure 2.3   Placebo effects in the context of a traditional medical model. In a medical model that ignores psychological processes, there are no adequate mechanisms to explain the operation of placebos.

One important development in our understanding of how psychological events—specifically, conditioned stimuli—can alter immune function has been the ingenious experiments conducted by Ader and Cohen (1993). In a prototype experiment, a group of rats was given a drug known to suppress the function of the immune system. Simultaneously with the drug, the animals were given saccharine in their water. Later, after the immune system had recovered, the animals were again exposed to the saccharine water, this time without the immunosuppressive drug. This resulted in a resuppression of immune function even though no active drug was present. To a rat, saccharine tastes different from sugar, so saccharine provided a novel taste sensation for these animals. Also, novel tastes are very salient stimuli for rats.

Ader and Cohen suggested that the saccharine-induced immunosuppression could be accounted for by a process of classical conditioning. In classical conditioning, we present a stimulus that has automatic effects on the body (such as food, which will lead to salivation in a dog), and we also present a stimulus unconnected with the original response (such as a bell or tone). Eventually the bell comes to elicit salivation, so we say the salivation has become conditioned to the sound. Figure 2.4 provides a diagram of the typical series of events in a Pavlovian conditioning experiment. In studies by Ader and his colleagues, we can think of the immunosuppressive drug as an unconditional stimulus (US), one that automatically produces an unconditional immunosuppressive response

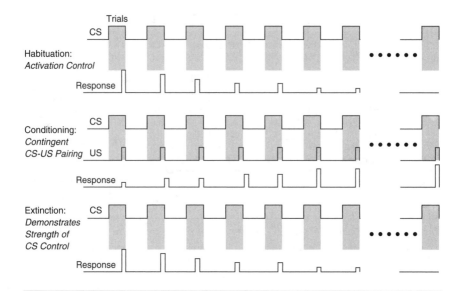

Figure 2.4 Pavlovian conditioning. In a typical Pavlovian, or classical, conditioning experiment, a stimulus such as food or shock is designated the unconditional stimulus because it evokes a response that is not dependent on other events. It is innately effective. The other stimulus, designated the conditional stimulus, is usually a sight or sound that has little or no effect other than to attract the momentary attention of the animal. Pairing the two stimuli ultimately changes the way the animal views and responds to the conditional stimulus so that the response to the conditional stimulus now mimics or anticipates the response to the unconditional stimulus.

(UR) due to its direct action on the system. We can also think of the saccharine as a conditional stimulus (CS), one that has no such effect on its own. Finally, we can see how the response to the saccharine alone became a conditioned response (CR) developed from the original UR associated with the CS-US pairing. Ader and Cohen's observations are a watershed in the science of immunology because they opened up the possibility that there could be unsuspected sources of influence on immune function and therefore on health.

The work of Ader and the discovery of the role of Pavlovian conditioning in immune system processes illustrate three points central to this book. First, the fact that Pavlovian conditioning can exert immunosuppressive effects means that an individual's experiential history places a definite stamp on the state of the body, both deleterious and beneficial.

Second, the experiment not only helps us understand psychological effects on immune function but also provides a clue as to the nature of some, if not all, placebo responses. We can think of the saccharine in Ader's studies as a kind of placebo, an inactive substance that acquired its powers through conditioning. Third, the taste of saccharine to the rat is really an *informational* stimulus. It had no power of its own, but it became a piece of information, a symbol, that something else might also happen—such as the administration of the immunosuppressive drug. Fourth, conditioning is not a special type of experience confined to the lab. Our entire lives are constantly emerging patterns of relationships with the environment. This pattern of relationships defines the meaning that events have for us, and conditioning provides a scientifically credible mechanism for how the world "gets under our skin," in the words of Anne Harrington (personal communication, 1995). The inactive saccharine, in other words, gained meaning because of the unique pairing with the drug, and the workings of the body were therefore altered. In this way, we can begin to think about how ideas and symbols may come to have power over our bodies.

The view that placebo responses are built on conditioned associations is not universally held. I find it satisfying to think that Pavlovian conditioning provides a mechanism for understanding how placebos might work, but not all placebo researchers agree that conditioning is the mechanism. Some researchers hold that if a given instance of a placebo response occurs because of the patient's expectancies, then a true placebo effect has occurred, but if conditioning caused the response, it is not a placebo effect at all but just another conditioned response (Ramsay & Woods, 2001). This controversy, like the placebo effect itself, illustrates the difficulty of clarifying mind-body issues in medicine. One wonders if Pavlovian conditioning is seen as a bad explanation for the placebo effect because it has a known mechanism but that expectancies are good explanations precisely because they don't have a known mechanism.

Expectancies may also be accompanied by conditioned responses, so the distinction may be arbitrary. Robert Rescorla (1988) discussed in a famous article how animals learn anticipatory responses during Pavlovian conditioning. After all, what was Pavlov's dog doing when he salivated to the sound of the bell, if not anticipating food? The conditioning explanation for placebos has the advantage of a parallel neurophysiological mechanism that gets us from symbols and ideas to physiological responses that affect the body. This is a powerful explanatory tool in favor of the conditioning model. The expectancy model, if it really is different from conditioning, has yet to be paired with an explicit neurophysiological process independent of conditioning. The lack of a physiological model for expectancies is certainly not a good argument in its favor. Again, the point of the discussion here is not to solve the placebo problem but to indicate the difficulties we face from a dualist perspective.

Cultural, Intrapersonal, and Physiological Influences in Coronary Heart Disease

A complex, chronic disease like coronary heart disease provides another instance of the limitations of a standard biomedical model and the uses of an expanded behavioral medicine model in understanding disease causation and treatment. In this example, there are even richer sources of behavioral input to the disease process and to its alleviation than in the case of infectious disease. What we call coronary heart disease, or coronary artery disease, is the result of the gradual accumulation of cholesterol-rich fatty plaques and thickened areas in the walls of the blood vessels that supply blood to the heart. This ultimately leads to an attenuated blood supply to the continually working heart muscle. The muscle receives too little oxygen, often causing the oppressive chest pain of angina pectoris. Occasionally a blood clot may form at the site of a thickened atherosclerotic lesion, completely blocking blood flow to the heart muscle downstream. This results in a heart attack, referred to by cardiologists as a myocardial infarction or MI.

Current treatments for this disease involve bypass grafts that circumvent the lesioned areas of the coronary artery by attachment of new vessels borrowed from other parts of the body; balloon angioplasty, which involves expanding the narrowed areas of a vessel by inserting a tiny balloon at the end of a catheter and inflating it at the restricted segment; angioplasty plus placement of an expandable mesh stent; or putting the patient on a low-cholesterol diet, sometimes supplemented by cholesterol-lowering drugs. Coronary artery bypass grafts and angioplasties were performed on more than 1.5 million men and women in the United States in 2000 (American Heart Association, 2003). All of these treatments are strictly within the traditional framework: They intervene in the pathogenic process at the tissue level.

Figure 2.5a shows a restricted, physicalist view of coronary artery disease and its treatment. In this view, the cause is a diet too high in cholesterol and saturated fats, perhaps helped along by a genetic predisposition to atherosclerosis. The cure is some combination of the therapies above. However, more recent evidence suggests that personal behaviors and cultural practices have much to do with the development of coronary

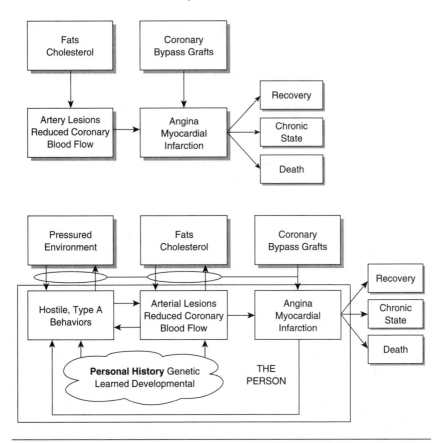

Figure 2.5   Traditional model of coronary artery disease (top) and an expanded model (bottom). Traditional treatments for coronary disease are shown as addressing the acute effects of the illness without addressing behavioral sources of the disorder. The expanded model indicates the potential for psychosocial causes, thereby indicating behavioral means of treatment.

heart disease. In the United States, we have a cultural practice of eating a diet high in animal fat and total calories. Further, some persons may aggravate the development of heart disease by regularly engaging in vigorous competitive behaviors accompanied by a hostile attitude. This constellation of extreme activity and hostile emotions, known as Type A behavior, may be associated with frequent elevations of blood pressure along with stress hormone secretion and the release of stored fat molecules into the bloodstream—all physiological processes that may accelerate lesion formation and growth.

With an expanded view of the disorder, depicted in Figure 2.5b, we can see the interplay of sociocultural, genetic, and personal habits in the etiology of the disease. In the expanded model, coronary heart disease does not have a simple unitary cause. Instead, a genetic heritage, a constellation of overt behaviors and emotional predispositions, and the specific cultural environment in which the behaviors and predispositions occur all increase or decrease disease risk. This expanded disease model not only allows for a more complete understanding of the development of coronary heart disease but also suggests insights into possible modes of therapy not possible under our more restricted model in Figure 2.5a. For example, it may be possible to provide cognitive and behavioral training to persons subject to frequent, emotionally intense, hostile interactions, thus lessening the destructive effects of blood pressure and catecholamine rises on the atherosclerotic vessels. In fact, such treatment in men who had experienced a first heart attack resulted in a significantly lower rate of second attacks compared to men who received only standard care (Friedman et al., 1986).

The dualistic view of ourselves that we have inherited via the Cartesian tradition leaves us with the problem of how psychosocial and sociocultural processes, which are by nature nonphysical, can act as causes of disease or as modes of treatment. Psychosocial and cultural processes are, at their root, informational. They shape our view of the world, our interpretations of social interactions, and ultimately our bodily responses. At the end of the book, we will consider an approach to this question that may help us dispense with distinctions between terms such as *physical, psychological,* and *sociocultural.*

Psychosocial Theories of Disease and Treatment

The examples above tell us that to understand all the causes of disease, and to consider the greatest possible range of treatments, we should recognize that neither the causes nor the cures are adequately described by a simple linear model. An expanded definition of disease might look like this: *a disorder of body functions or systems arising from physiological, psychophysiological, or sociocultural malfunctioning.*

Several authors have considered the role of psychological and sociocultural processes in treatment (see, e.g., Elstein & Bordage, 1979). We may consider a revised view of treatment, taking into account some traditional and nontraditional questions:

1. Who is being treated? The patient's psychological makeup, learning history, and cultural background may be important elements in developing a plan of treatment.

2. What is the specific disease state? Accurate diagnosis is crucial to successful treatment.

3. What factors limit treatment alternatives? Not all treatments are feasible at all times.

4. What is the social environment? This may facilitate some treatments and limit the uses of others.

5. What is the specific form of treatment? Clearly, all other considerations aside, the treatment must ultimately interact appropriately with the disease process at a physical level.

6. What is the therapist's psychological makeup? The success of treatment may be influenced by the practitioner's attitudes.

7. What is the mode of therapy? The form of therapy must be tailored to meet the restrictions imposed by 1 through 6 above.

8. What is the goal of treatment? Given any disease state, the goals of treatment will be based on realistic considerations of 1 through 7 above.

The Foundation of Behavioral Medicine

Behavioral medicine involves the study of how sociocultural and mind-brain processes can influence the health of an individual. It seeks to identify ways that maladaptive behaviors, states of mind, or cultural practices may impair health and how these same processes can be used to improve it.

In an influential chapter on behavioral medicine titled "The Brain as a Health Care System," Gary Schwartz (1979) argued that general systems theory offers a way to conceptualize the role of the mind-brain in health and disease. Systems theory describes how simple and complex systems are regulated and how they maintain that regulation when threatened with disruption. Schwartz pointed out that the brain is engaged constantly in hierarchically integrating information to regulate bodily functions, such as respiration. By *hierarchically*, we mean that bodily functions have several layers of control, each layer being modified by the one above. The layered-control concept provides a way of thinking about how our higher brain activities, such as thoughts and emotions, can act on lower centers to alter bodily functions. In calling the brain a health care system, Schwartz acknowledged that the brain ultimately plays the topmost role in regulating physiological systems and is essential in maintaining the health of the body not only through physiological regulation but through emotions, thoughts, and behaviors. Finally, the brain interprets and assimilates social and cultural information, and its interpretations in turn influence the workings of the body.

Schwartz proposed a five-stage model to illustrate these processes:

1. The organism and the environment are involved in a two-way dialogue. We receive information from our external environment and continuously modify that environment by our actions. For example, if the room is cold, we might get up and raise the thermostat or put on a sweater.

2. The mind-brain integrates information from the external and internal environments and uses these two sources of information to determine regulation of the somatic organs. When we are cold, we might shiver to increase our body temperature.

3. The somatic organs alter their function to adapt to external and internal demands according to activity determined by the brain. In this way, they function to maintain an optimal balance for the body's internal environment. This topic will receive primary attention in Chapters 3, 4, and 5, which deal with the concept of stress, physiological regulation, and responses to physical and psychological challenges.

4. In carrying out its regulatory role, the brain makes heavy use of *interoceptive* information, the inputs the brain receives from the viscera, muscles, and joints. For example, in the short-term regulation of blood pressure, the brainstem receives constant input from the baroreceptors located in the aorta and carotid arteries. Deviations from normal pressure lead to rapid changes in the heart's rate and force of contraction. This allows sudden pressure changes to be compensated for almost instantly and automatically. These processes happen automatically without our awareness.

5. Finally, it is possible for the brain to use external sources of information to regulate the body. An everyday example is that we may look at the temperature setting on a thermostat to adjust it to ensure a comfortable environment in our home or office. A more subtle and striking example of information-based regulation is the process of *biofeedback*. In biofeedback, a bodily function normally not accessible to our awareness, such as blood pressure, is displayed visually or auditorally to allow conscious access to the momentary state of that function. By this means, it becomes possible with practice to change the function for

short periods: for example, to raise or lower blood pressure by altering processes controlling it, such as heart rate. Biofeedback therefore provides another information channel for the brain to have access to and alter processes in the body, at least temporarily. (Biofeedback probably cannot permanently lower blood pressure in a person with hypertension.) Biofeedback can also allow patients who suffer from muscle tension to develop conscious awareness of episodes of tension and to recognize which muscles are tensing up. After several sessions of feedback, the person may become able to do this outside the clinic and take steps to relax the appropriate muscle groups before they become painful. This is a simple but effective technique for gaining awareness to regulate the state of our bodies.

Both Schwartz's ideas on the brain's regulation of body processes and the expanded disease model shown in Figure 2.2 place a significant emphasis on the role of information received by the brain to alter the functions of the body. Schwartz makes the important point that there is no fundamental difference between the interoceptive information the brain uses in its normal regulation of the body and the information it receives from outside as determined by the behaviors of the individual or by the cultural environment. We will return to the concept of hierarchical control by the brain in considering autonomic regulation in Chapter 4 and in our description of central nervous integrations of psychological stress responses in Chapters 6 and 7.

Summary

In this chapter, we described how the mind-body dualism of Descartes affected the Western view of physiology and medicine and in turn led to an unnecessarily narrow view of disease and treatment. We described a revised model of disease in which thoughts and emotions can be major elements in treatment. By acknowledging the role of psychosocial and socio-cultural processes, behavioral medicine expands our ways of thinking about the influences on health and disease.

We said in Chapter 1 that our dualistic view of humans as having two fundamentally different natures, physical and spiritual, leaves us few conceptual tools to help us understand and explain how the mind alters the body. As a result, we do not yet have a generally accepted, scientifically grounded model for appreciating how thoughts and emotions affect health. To take this abstract discussion of behavioral medicine closer to reality, we must do two things. First, we must confront the obstacles to our thinking that are conditioned by our intellectual heritage. For this reason, I have sketched the history of our dualistic model of ourselves. If we continue to think of physical processes and mental or psychological functions as being in separate realms, we will have a much more difficult time envisioning how our state of health and disease are conditioned by our thoughts, feelings, and actions. We will return to this topic in our last chapter and consider some ways of further advancing our understanding. Second, we must address the mechanisms by which the brain controls the body and find the linkages between ideas and regulatory processes. In a sense, we need to follow the steps between the idea and the bodily function if we are to answer our primary question of how an idea can come to have power over our bodies: how mental stress can affect our health. Fortunately, progress is being made on both these fronts. In Chapters 9 and 10, we will present recent models of chronic stress that allow us to think about the products of negative emotions and persistent feelings of distress as causes of changes in the body and brain that may be health impairing. There are also recent models showing how early nurturing and beneficial environments may improve stress reactivity and long-term health in adulthood. These advances in research point toward future areas of study that will have a considerable impact on our thinking about the mind and the body.

Further Reading

Foss, L., & Rothenberg, K. (1988). *The second medical revolution.* Boston: Shambhala.
Schwartz, G. (1979). The brain as a health care system. In G. C. Stone, F. Cohen, & N. E. Adler (Eds.), *Health psychology: A handbook* (pp. 549–571). San Francisco: Jossey-Bass.

Two primary sources for material covered in this chapter. Together, they provide a broad view of the relationship of behavioral medicine to traditional medicine.

Sarafino, E. P. (2001). *Health psychology: Biopsychosocial interactions* (4th ed.). New York: John Wiley.

An excellent standard text that describes the biopsychosocial model from a behavioral medicine perspective.

Harrington, A. (1997). *The placebo effect: An interdisciplinary exploration.* Cambridge, MA: Harvard University Press.

An important work on the placebo phenomenon, viewed broadly from the perspective of several disciplines.

3

History of the
Concept of Stress

In the first two chapters, we asked how ideas could alter the workings of the body. We described how the mind-body problem has created barriers to understanding how the brain's functioning could be altered by what we perceive, think, and feel. We began to make a case for considering the role of the brain in altering physiological function for better or worse. Our argument can be summarized as follows: The brain is how we make contact with the external environment. The interactions are ultimately *regulatory* in nature. The regulatory process seeks to preserve normal, healthy functioning. We could say that the brain's primary purpose is to provide the highest level of behavioral and physiological regulation, dedicated to maintaining health, fitness, and reproductive success. Because the central nervous system is dedicated to sustaining life and coping with external threats, it must be seen as the primary focus of a behavioral medicine. Therefore, we will address the question of stress responses as potential modifiers of health within a behavioral medicine framework.

The dictionary defines *stress* as a bodily or mental tension resulting from factors that tend to alter an existent equilibrium (*Merriam-Webster's Collegiate Dictionary*, 1993). Note that the definition has two elements. First, there is a tension, presumably caused by some force pulling on the system. Second, the tension is a threat to the normal equilibrium of the system. These two elements tell us that stress is an active process that involves an action on the system that threatens its equilibrium. It is assumed that the tension may cause harm unless some process of compensation reduces the disequilibrium to a baseline level or the cause is removed. It follows that a *stressor* is a stimulus event that challenges the integrity, or health, of the body (*Merriam-Webster's Collegiate Dictionary*, 1993), and a *stress response* is the body's compensatory reaction to that challenge.

The notion of compensation is a third element in our understanding of stress: There is a force, a resulting tension, and some compensation, without which the force would do harm to the system. The tension would thus seem to result from (a) the size of the challenging force and (b) the need for the system to compensate for the challenge. The greater the challenge and the less the compensation, the greater the tension and the potential for damage to the system. The state of stress is ended when the tension is removed by compensating for the stressor and eventually eliminating it. For example, consider how we might react to cold. Because we need to maintain an adequate body temperature, exposure to cold is a threat to our integrity and perhaps to our life. In a minor case, we may experience a mild degree of threat to our well-being if the office is a bit colder than we would like. The compensation required of us may be no more than setting the thermostat or putting on a sweater. If we do either of these things, we are comfortably warm, and the threat of chills has been eliminated. What happens in more extreme circumstances? We face a more severe challenge if we are at a football game on a snowy day with the wrong clothing on. The demand is greater, the necessary compensation is greater, and if we can't find some warm clothes, the difference between the demand and our ability to compensate determines a much more severe stress state that is potentially damaging. Figure 3.1 illustrates this point. The three degrees of stress show arrows of different lengths that go from the compensation to the demand imposed by the environment. The greater the demand, and the more compensation that is required, the greater the state of stress. We might say that the stress results from the demand and that compensatory capability is a function of the distance that has to be covered in reducing the threat to zero. The greater the demand and the less ability we have to reduce it, the greater will be our state of stress.

The dictionary definition also mentions bodily *or* mental tensions. This implies that we can distinguish between stresses that are physical and those that are psychological in origin. We think of physical stressors as ones that pose a direct threat to our physical well-being. Cold is one such stressor, and so are heat, infection, and toxic substances. Psychological stressors are events that challenge our safety, not because they

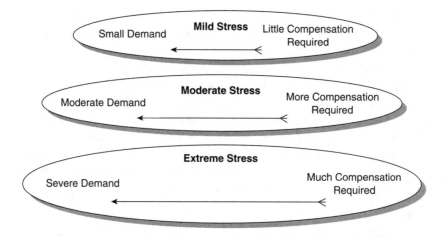

Figure 3.1   The state of stress is illustrated by the amount of demand posed by the environment and the amount of compensation required to keep the system within homeostatic limits. The length of the line connecting the demand and the compensation indicates the extent to which the system must use energy and compensatory resources to balance the demand. The greater this is, the greater the amount of stress on the system. The stress will be maintained until the threat is eliminated. Failure to eliminate the threat may result in damage to the system.

are physically dangerous, but because of our thoughts, perceptions, and interpretations. We may find that a major personal disappointment—say, failing to get into graduate school—causes great emotional distress. Or the sound of footsteps on a dark street may provoke a feeling of terror. The disappointment may evoke physical sensations of sadness, lethargy, or even tears of grief. The footsteps may result in fear, along with a racing heart and rapid breathing. In both cases, our physiological responses start out as thoughts and interpretations, mental events that are not in fact physically threatening and are not things at all. The emotions and physiological responses arise because of our interpretation of the event and its perceived meaning in terms of our well-being. We will explore the process of psychological stress further in Chapter 5, where we will consider how ideas can affect the body.

There have been four milestones in the development of our understanding of stress. First was the recognition that the *internal environment* of the body must be protected from the *external environment* in order to sustain the living cells and tissues. Second was the formulation of the concept of *homeostasis,* or regulation of the stability of the internal environment by an organized system of controls. Third was the recognition that during states of stress a consistent pattern of *nonspecific responses,* the so-called general adaptation syndrome, is called forth to resist the potential damage posed by the challenge. Fourth was the idea that long-term stresses exact an adaptive cost, known as an *allostatic load,* that may impair health. A review of the history of the development of the stress concept indicates that we are still squarely at the crux of the Cartesian dilemma. Although we know much more about systemic regulation and stress responses than we did in the past, we still have difficulty integrating the idea of psychological causes into a model of physiological stress responses.

Claude Bernard and the Concept of the Internal Environment

Certain ideas have such a hold on the imagination that they appear again and again in different forms throughout history. One such idea is the belief that living things are special and have a privileged status in the material world. Descartes's ideas profoundly influenced the development of an empirical science of living things. Although even he reserved a special place for the soul in the workings of the brain, he saw that living things are material in nature and can be studied as we might study nonliving things.

However, in the early part of the 19th century, the school of vitalism reopened this issue by arguing that living things had special status in the order of things. Vitalism is the idea that living things are driven by a nonphysical life force (*élan vital*) that does not obey "physicochemical" laws. The vitalists held that the vital force was responsible for making living things different from inanimate matter. We may think of the vital force as a variant of what Gilbert Ryle called the "Ghost in the Machine." According to vitalist doctrine, the presence of the nonmaterial life force made it impossible to study living organisms by a reductionistic strategy: A study of the subcomponents would disrupt the vital force, leaving the results of such study invalid.

An opposing viewpoint was taken by Claude Bernard (1813–1878), the great French founder of physiology, who argued that living things are amenable to a reductionistic research strategy (Bernard, 1865/1961). Bernard's primary task in arguing the scientific side of this debate was to explain away the apparent mystery by which some invisible force supposedly moved the machinery of the body. He started by using the analogy of how we might study a steam engine if we had never seen one before. Without careful examination of how the engine used energy to produce steam and convert the pressure of the steam to mechanical forces propelling the wheels, it would be easy to conclude that such machines possessed a mysterious internal force responsible for their movements. (Descartes had used similar mechanical analogies.) However, argued Bernard, it would be obvious to any mid-19th-century observer that a steam engine was in fact a machine whose actions were completely determined by the laws of chemistry and mechanics. The pressure of steam moved the train's inanimate metal parts, the arms that caused the wheels to turn. The whole process was started by the combustion of coal or wood that liberated stored energy to boil the water. The mystery of the self-propelled iron horse was no mystery at all if one followed step-by-step the liberation of the stored energy, its transformation to steam, and the levers that turned the wheels, all demonstrable using reductionistic methods. Bernard thus argued that the mechanical determinism associated with living things was in principle no different from that of the steam engine.

Because Bernard's primary challenge was to remove the mystery of movement possessed by living things, he needed to deal with the problem of how living organisms could move themselves even when no external force was seen to be acting upon them. He made his case by arguing that living things had an *internal environment* that caused their behavior. Beginning with very simple animals, he showed that one-celled organisms depend on a supportive external environment and are able to maintain themselves only if the correct external factors, such as moisture, temperature, oxygenation, and nutrients, are available from the medium in which they live. Such animals are not capable of maintaining themselves independent of their external environments. Their behaviors and metabolic functions clearly result from chemical and physical interactions with their surroundings and are highly responsive to any changes in external conditions. As a result of this dependency, the causal factors related to the maintenance of life are most obvious in these simple creatures.

In contrast, more highly developed organisms have greater autonomy from their environments. Mammals, for example, have an internal circulation that duplicates the conditions of the external medium surrounding one-celled life forms. They can regulate temperature, acid-base balance of the blood, oxygenation of the cells, and a supply of nutrients by regulating the conditions of their blood supplies in the face of changing external conditions. Thus, they have the outward appearance of being autonomous and possessing a hidden life force. However, the appearance of such a life force is an illusion. Complex animals are no less deterministically dependent on the conditions in which they find themselves. Viewed at the cellular level, they too are highly responsive to any change in the conditions of the internal environment.

Therefore, Bernard held that the functions of complex living organisms are determined by both the external environment and the internal environment. He noted that the maintenance of life was critically dependent on responses that keep the internal environment constant in the face of a changing external environment. Such responses, obeying the chemical and physical laws governing biological systems, create the illusion of a life force that drives the otherwise inert-appearing machinery of the body. Bernard's key idea, that physical challenges to the integrity of an organism provoke responses to counteract those threats, is the foundation of our modern concept of stress and stress responses, although the word *stress* was first used in this way by Walter Cannon.

Walter Cannon and the Concept of Homeostasis

The next major figure in the development of our present ideas about stress and physiological regulation is Walter Cannon, the first professor of physiology at Harvard University. Cannon (1929) researched the specific mechanisms of responding to changes in the external environment while allowing for optimum bodily function. He began with Bernard's idea that we are immersed in an internalized fluid environment and that we have evolved mechanisms to keep this environment constant to support our cells and organs. He termed the process of maintaining internal stability in the face of environmental change *homeostasis*. This concept was useful in focusing the attention of physiologists and psychologists on the collective mechanisms by which the state of the internal environment was maintained in an optimal range. Cannon's work dealt with the specialized sensory nerves that communicate the state of the body to the brain. He also studied which areas of the brain had the structures needed to detect these internal states and invoke the proper compensatory responses. His work therefore contributed much to the foundation of knowledge on the workings of the autonomic nervous system and the regulation of the body.

Cannon's thinking was not confined to the mechanisms of physical challenges. Although he was first and foremost a physiologist who studied the autonomic and endocrine responses that regulated metabolism, he was well aware that we also respond to deviations from normal by invoking behavioral changes to alter the impact of the environment. Anticipating the concept of psychological stress, he also concerned himself with the impact on the person of psychologically meaningful stimuli, as seen in the example of the jealous wife with the heart symptoms that we quoted in Chapter 1 (Cannon, 1935).

Bernard and Cannon together contributed greatly to the philosophy of medical science and to the development of the concept of stress. Bernard's recognition that the cells of our bodies are in contact with an internal environment that must be held constant led to the further recognition that there had to be a hierarchy of control mechanisms to compensate for changes from normal. We noted in Chapter 2 that to account fully for the ways in which persons maintain health, we had to develop a model in which there were successive layers of control capable of managing the system during states of disease. Cannon studied the physical mechanisms we use to maintain homeostasis, but he also saw that loss of good health could result from dysregulation of the system at the level of psychological and sociocultural functioning.

Our approach to behavioral medicine therefore begins with the physiological mechanisms by which environmental alterations are countered in order to maintain life, and we will later examine the parallel effects of psychological challenges to our well-being and how these too result in regulatory changes to meet perceived threats. Though Cannon was the first to use the term *stress* in terms of the demands placed on the body and the body's responses, it was the work of another pioneering researcher, Hans Selye, that brought the concept of stress to the attention of the world's medical community.

Hans Selye and the General Adaptation Syndrome

The work of Hans Selye consolidated the concept of stress, and he is recognized as the father of stress research. Following Cannon, he became the first to invoke systematically the concept of stress as a means of understanding physiological regulatory responses to threats to the organism. The two concepts of homeostasis and stress have since provided powerful organizing principles allowing numerous researchers to consider threats to our well-being and the variety of ways we can respond to them.

On the basis of his early work, Selye (1936, 1956) became interested in how animals reacted to various challenges to their homeostasis, including heat, cold, infection, and toxic substances. His major contribution was in noticing that all such challenges called forth in the experimental animals a consistent pattern of response, including a decrease in the size of the thymus gland and other immune system organs; ulcers in the gastrointestinal tract; and enlargement of the adrenal glands. Because application of severe stressors always produced this set of changes, Selye argued that it constituted the universal core of the stress response pattern, and he termed it the *general adaptation syndrome*. Selye also observed that because stressors had individual characteristics, specific responses were called into play to meet their unique features. The full pattern of the responses to a stressor therefore consisted of a central, nonspecific adaptation syndrome plus the specific responses that would address the particular event at hand. This basic formulation has stood as a solid foundation for the interpretation of numerous studies since its first publication.

The general adaptation syndrome was a process that unfolded over time. Selye identified three stages by which this constellation of nonspecific and specific responses worked toward the organism's survival. The first was the *alarm reaction*, during which the stressor first registered itself on the system and the organism began to mount its response. The second stage Selye referred to as the *stage of resistance*, during which the organism produced the necessary metabolic changes to sustain life and would maintain this compensatory reaction as long as the requisite stores of fuel and biochemical substrates were available. This resistance would persist for as long as necessary, sometimes for days, until the stressor was overcome or the animal was no longer able to mount the defense. The third and final phase was the *stage of exhaustion*, leading to the ultimate death of the animal under study.

Selye recognized that the stress response was adaptive because it sought to preserve the life of the threatened organism. But he also recognized that there was a cost to the animal in mounting a stress response. The three components of the general adaptation syndrome are actually manifestations of tissue pathology due to severe and prolonged activation caused by mounting the stress response. Selye's studies showed that during the phase of resistance to one stressor, the animal's ability to withstand a second, even a milder, challenge was impaired. Further, he pointed out that repeated exposure to moderate stressors could actually increase the organism's ability to withstand more prolonged and severe exposure to the same stressor. Athletic coaches make use of this idea by using frequent, moderate episodes of physical training to expand athletes' capacities to exercise harder and longer in preparation for the stress of competition.

Therefore, stress responses have long-term consequences, some beneficial and some harmful. The focus on long-term effects drew attention to the nature of the changes the organism might experience and under what circumstances. This set of effects was encapsulated in the most recent conceptual addition to our understanding of stress, the idea of *allostasis*.

The Concept of Allostasis

Cannon introduced the term *homeostasis* to encapsulate the totality of the processes we use to counteract threats to our well-being. The concept of homeostasis may lead us to imagine that once balance has been restored, the organism returns to some sort of resting or prestress state in which energetic demands once again are reduced to minimum and no extra costs are incurred to keep us alive and well. In many cases, this may be so. However, Sterling and Eyer (1988) insightfully observed that homeostasis could also be achieved in a way that exerted a continuing cost to the system. Consider the case of a person who is left in the cold and who can maintain a normal body temperature, but only by violent shivering and vigorous movement. In this case, the adaptation the person has made to the cold is costly and highly energy consuming. Sterling and Eyer coined the term *allostasis* to capture the idea that when a demand has not been removed or neutralized, maintaining homeostasis may be a source of ongoing wear and tear on the system. Without using the term itself, Selye was aware of the costs of adaptation: He noted that the resistance phase of the general adaptation syndrome could not be indefinitely maintained and that the resources of the animal would eventually be exhausted (Selye, 1956). Cannon (1935) similarly noted the adaptive cost of maintaining homeostasis and the ultimate decline in the ability to maintain the adaptation. Selye and Cannon were thinking here of moderately long-lasting but not chronic stressors. Since Sterling and Eyer's introduction of the concept, Bruce McEwen and Elliot Stellar (1993) have made considerable use of it and expanded its initial formulation. In particular, they have invoked the idea of an *allostatic load,* encapsulating the idea of the costs of maintaining homeostasis in the face of continuing challenges that may go on for months or years.

The concept of allostasis gains special utility when we take into account more gentle, persistent, and less life-threatening stresses such as the anxiety and aggravation of caring for an infirm and elderly loved one or the physiological costs of coping with a nonlethal but chronic infection. These lesser stresses may be suspected of causing long-term damage to health, even if the short-term effect is negligible, because they exert a constant bias or demand on the system. The ongoing demand competes for coping resources and reduces the ability of the person to cope psychologically or physiologically with new demands that may be imposed by other stressors encountered in daily life. This idea has gained currency in the stress field since 1993 and seems likely to become a useful addition to it. Clinicians and researchers are beginning to find allostasis an effective concept that captures specific aspects of the costs of long-term adaptation to chronic stressors and leads to a productive way to phrase research questions and summarize their findings.

Stress Responses Are a Part of Normal Physiological Regulation

Because stress responses are often accompanied by negative emotions, we may tend to think of stress responses as bad, somehow to be avoided, indeed, abnormal. But there is a sense in which our ability to have stress reactions represents one part of the normal process of physiological regulation. It follows from the discussion above that all living things need regulatory mechanisms to keep their internal environments within limits in order to resist destruction by outside forces. Also, the concept of stress is qualitative. It is unclear when a small perturbation in our environment calls on a small adjustment in our systemic function or when the challenge is potentially life threatening.

We said above that stress is any source of disruption in the orderly workings of the body. We might rephrase that to say that a *stressor* is any severe challenge or threat to the normal processes or integrated function of a living thing. The response of the organism to that threat is the *stress response*. A threat exists when the environment begins to move beyond the range of normal for the system or the organism. So a small change in the temperature of our living room is not necessarily a stressor, although it may result in some response. In contrast, being locked out of the house for an hour or more on a freezing evening might evoke not only severe physiological adjustments but major behavioral ones as well, including breaking back into the house by any means necessary. The magnitude of the stress therefore depends on a dynamic relationship between the stressor and the compensatory processes.

All biological systems are organized to respond to the environment. They can tolerate a range of environmental conditions, and they must compensate for each of these, within their limitations, to prevent damage or death. At some point, severe enough environmental circumstances will result in complete cessation of systems-level function (death). Stress implies a level of challenge severe enough to require major or prolonged readjustments to meet the challenge. If compensation is perfect and rapid, little or no stress occurs in the system. If compensation is imperfect or inadequate, the stress effect is larger and may be threatening to life or health.

In Chapter 2, we noted that adjustments can occur hierarchically and involve several levels in systems organization: cells, organs, systems, and still higher levels of integration involving overt behavior influenced by ideas and cultural norms. As one level in the system is no longer able to compensate fully or adequately for the environmental challenge, higher levels come into play. Ultimately these higher controls may include becoming aware that a problem exists, evaluating the problem, considering courses of action, making behavioral adjustments to compensate for the imbalance, and perhaps actually altering the environment itself. So to return to our example of exposure to the cold, we can think of mild shivering as a systems response to a slightly cool living room, and we can think of breaking into a house when one is locked out on a cold night as a severe behavioral adjustment, both of which have the ultimate purpose of returning our body temperature to normal. All levels in the system are therefore capable of contributing to stress responses in the service of the individual's survival.

People differ in how responsive they are to environmental threats and how they compensate. This issue of individual differences will arise in Chapter 10 when we think about stress and disease predisposition.

Summary

Our current understanding of stress and its effects is based on the idea that the delicate machinery of the body has to have a relatively constant internal environment to work in. To do so, it must have a way to protect itself and maintain homeostasis when outside conditions change undesirably. Multiple control systems must operate to maintain homeostasis. When the threat is severe enough, we may have to mount a full-scale stress response to meet and overcome the challenge. However, the use of these powerful physiological controls may be damaging if the state of stress is very severe or very prolonged. The allostatic load imposed on the system by maintaining homeostasis when demand cannot be eliminated may therefore impair long-term health. The next chapter will discuss the specific control mechanisms the body uses to maintain homeostasis.

Further Reading

Bernard, C. (1961). *An introduction to the study of experimental medicine* (H. C. Greene, Trans.). New York: Collier Books. (Original work published 1865)

A highly readable and interesting discussion of early concepts in physiology, with emphasis on the epistemological groundwork that determined the development of biology from that time to the present.

Cannon, W. B. (1929). *Bodily changes in pain, hunger, fear, and rage* (2nd ed.). New York: Appleton.

Walter Cannon's most important work, this book can surprise the reader with its sophistication and scientific clarity.

Cannon, W. B. (1935). Stresses and strains of homeostasis (Mary Scott Newbold Lecture). *American Journal of Medical Sciences, 189,* 1–14.

Cannon's first use of the term *homeostasis.*

Selye, H. (1956). *The stress of life.* New York: McGraw-Hill.

Selye's most complete statement of his views on stress. A classic in the stress field.

Fink, G. (Ed.). (2000). *The encyclopedia of stress* (Vols. 1–3). New York: Academic Press.

An extensive encyclopedia with specialized articles on every aspect of stress, from biology to prevention.

4

Homeostatic Regulation

Understanding homeostatic regulation during stress requires understanding the mechanisms the body uses to maintain homeostatic function during more normal periods. We can divide homeostatic regulation into five layers:

1. *Organs and their local reflexes.* Organs can regulate their own functions with systems of built-in reflexes that need no higher level of control to function effectively.

2. *Autonomic and endocrine messengers.* The autonomic nervous system and the endocrine system form two channels of descending communication from the central nervous system to the individual organs.

3. *Brainstem regulation.* The brainstem regulates autonomic outputs to the organs through a complex network of reflex centers.

4. *Hypothalamic integrations.* The hypothalamus regulates endocrine messengers to the body. It also coordinates actions of the brainstem autonomic nuclei.

5. *Inputs from higher brain centers.* Brain areas above the hypothalamus have inputs from the external world and can use this information to form emotions, memories, and awareness. These higher processes can then alter the activities of the hypothalamus and brainstem.

This system of controls is schematized in Figure 4.1.

This chapter covers the first four of these levels of control. Chapter 5 discusses the concept of psychological stress and its similarities to and

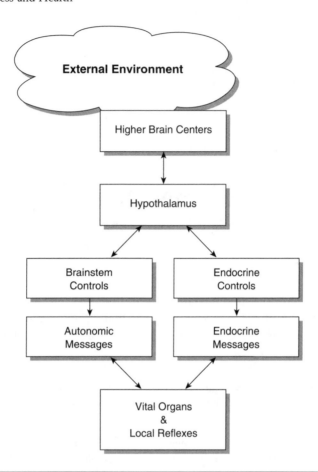

Figure 4.1   Schematic of controls over organic function. The diagram indicates that individual organs have self-regulating capacity. This self-regulation is determined by internal reflexes and the actions of autonomic ganglia located in or near them. Local regulation is modulated in turn by descending influences from the autonomic nervous system, the brainstem, the hypothalamus, and higher centers in the central nervous system.

differences from physical stress. Chapter 6 addresses the influences imposed by the higher brain centers, their integration with emotions and behavior, and their effects on stress mechanisms. Chapter 7 is devoted to a further discussion of endocrine regulation. Therefore, we will spend four chapters developing an overview of how autonomic and endocrine responses operate normally, how they respond to physical threats to homeostasis, and how the workings of the system can be altered by psychological stimulation.

A Hierarchy of Homeostatic Controls

At the bottom of the hierarchical system of controls shown in Figure 4.1 are vital organs and their local reflexes. The vital organs have intrinsic reflexive control mechanisms that allow them to operate without further assistance when external conditions are constant. In addition, the individual organs have reflex loops to the ganglia of the autonomic nervous system and the spinal cord to aid in this local regulation. The organs and their simple reflexes are able to respond to strictly local needs. However, there are times when the organs alone cannot alter their function to meet rapid changes in demand or to coordinate their functions across organs. At such times, two parallel systems of communication from the central nervous system regulate organ function, the autonomic nervous system and the endocrine system. These systems are regulated and coordinated by the brainstem and the hypothalamus. The brainstem directly controls the autonomic nervous system. The hypothalamus controls the endocrine system, coordinates actions of the autonomic and endocrine systems, and has motor areas that store specific programs encoding survival-related behaviors. Because the autonomic nervous system and endocrine system communicate to multiple organs, they can produce complex coordination that goes beyond the capability of individual organs in adjusting to meet changes in external conditions. Finally, the mechanisms of the brainstem and hypothalamus cannot meet every kind of need. There are times when external sensory inputs and behavioral responses involving the skeletal motor system are needed to cope with emergencies and ensure survival. At these times, higher brain centers have to be brought into the picture. These centers include the limbic system and the cerebral cortex. Their functioning is particularly important during times of stress in shaping the outputs that are generated by lower systems.

This hierarchical organization of controls has the virtue of allowing local processes to proceed on their own, leaving our limited conscious processing ability free for immediate tasks. But sometimes it may be necessary for local activity to become coordinated with the functions of other organs to achieve a common purpose. For example, during intense exercise, the actions of the heart and blood vessels may need to be integrated for maximum performance. In this case, endocrine and integrated autonomic controls may come into play. At still other times, the person's awareness may need to be brought to bear on the entire system to meet particular long-term needs. For example, the person who is jogging may recall that the exercise session has to end now because of family responsibilities, so the lower autonomic centers and the exercising muscles receive the signal to slow down and head for home. In this case, the highest level of control over homeostasis is exerted by the cerebral cortex.

Intrinsic Control Mechanisms

Each vital organ or organ system is capable of regulating its own function in response to slowly changing environmental demands. An example of the ability of an organ to regulate itself is the way the heart controls its own pumping action. First, the heart regulates its rate of contraction by its internal pacemaker, the sinoatrial node. This pacemaker node, located in the heart's atrial muscle, is a collection of specialized neurons that fire rhythmically and at a steady rate. By itself, the human heart will beat steadily at about 110 beats per minute unless told to do otherwise by the autonomic nervous system or an endocrine messenger. Similarly, the force of the heart's contraction is regulated internally by the Frank-Starling mechanism. The Frank-Starling response is a result of the inherent property of the cardiac muscle to contract more effectively when stretched to a greater degree. As a result, the heart responds in proportion to the amount of blood returning to it from the systemic circulation. When blood returning to the heart increases, the atrial chambers of the heart fill more completely before each beat. This more effective filling of the ventricles creates more wall stretch. The muscle fibers are consequently put under more tension, resulting in a more vigorous contraction on that beat. The left ventricle therefore empties more completely, producing more effective flow into the aorta. In this manner, the heart keeps up with the flow demands placed on it by the systemic circulation. Finally, the heart's four chambers and system for conducting muscular contraction are physically designed to cause this complex organ to automatically contract in a coordinated manner. More detail on the actions of the heart can be found in Guyton and Hall's (2000, chs. 9 and 10) textbook on human physiology.

The existence of these intrinsic cardiac controls means that if the heart is deprived of its autonomic innervation and its endocrine inputs, it will continue to supply blood to all the tissues of the body. It will maintain adequate blood flow completely on its own and without external control—as long as conditions remain constant. Unfortunately, if the individual possessing this functionally isolated heart were to do something so simple as to stand up suddenly, blood would move down into the legs and the amount of blood returning to the heart would drop precipitously. The heart would be uninformed that the state of the organism had changed and would be unable to rapidly increase its output of blood to respond to this brief, routine demand. Similarly, the blood vessels would not compensate for the sudden redistribution of the blood to the legs. As a result, the person might faint from a rapid drop in blood supply to the brain. So although the heart's intrinsic controls can deal with constant conditions, such as when the person is sitting or lying down, rapid changes in demand must be met by additional controls supplied by endocrine and autonomic inputs.

Autonomic and Endocrine Controls Over Homeostasis

Walter Cannon (1935) proposed that homeostasis was maintained by a system of negative feedback loops. Negative feedback is the most common form of regulation in the autonomic and endocrine systems. As its name implies, this mechanism acts by detecting the state of a controlled activity, comparing that state to a set point, and exerting an opposite influence if the function departs from the set point. Negative feedback describes how a thermostat shuts off a furnace when the room temperature has risen above the level set at the thermostat. Maintaining homeostasis through negative feedback requires that the brainstem and hypothalamus receive information about the state of the bodily organs and return commands to those same organs by way of the autonomic nervous system and endocrine messengers.

The autonomic and endocrine systems are both motor systems with similarities to and differences from the more familiar skeletal motor system. The skeletal motor system is a conscious and voluntary system. It has sensory nerves that give the brain information about the position and motion of the limbs. These nerves project to sensory areas of the cerebral cortex, and these cortical sensory projections allow us to be aware of where our limbs are and what they are doing. Similarly, the skeletal motor nerves run from motor areas of the cerebral cortex directly to individual muscle fiber bundles to command their movements. Therefore, we have voluntary control over our movements. The sensory and motor nerves are located directly in the cerebral cortex, so we are conscious of the position of our limbs and have voluntary control of our movements. One motor nerve fiber reaches a single fiber bundle, leading to very precise control of the target muscle by a given nerve.

The autonomic nervous system also has sensory and motor nerves. However, its sensory nerves do not rise to the level of the cerebral cortex, and its motor nerves originate in the brainstem. As a result, we have limited awareness of the state of our vital organs. Similarly, we have very little control over them. For the most part, they act entirely on their own. Therefore, we say that the autonomic nervous system acts *autonomously*, without conscious awareness or voluntary control. The autonomic nerve fibers reaching a target organ or tissue are highly branched, and the smooth muscle cells themselves are highly interconnected. This results in more widespread responses on the part of the effectors than is true in the skeletal motor system.

The following description of the autonomic nervous system is necessarily brief. A highly readable, well-illustrated presentation is provided in Kandel, Schwartz, and Jessel (2000).

Three Autonomic Divisions

The autonomic nervous system, shown in Figure 4.2, controls the vital organs by way of three anatomically and functionally distinct branches: the *sympathetic nervous system*, the *parasympathetic nervous system*, and the *enteric nervous system*.

Each division of the autonomic nervous system has sensory nerves and four major response components. The sensory nerves run from the organs through the ganglia and from there to the brainstem. The response components are:

1. *Descending autonomic fibers* and *preganglionic fibers.* Fibers originating in the hypothalamus and brainstem autonomic nuclei descend by way of the intermediolateral cell column of the spinal cord. Here these descending fibers leave the intermediolateral cell column and give rise to preganglionic fibers that exit at specific levels of the spinal column and travel to their respective ganglia. Preganglionic fibers are therefore ones that exit the spinal cord and travel to autonomic ganglia located outside the spinal cord. The hypothalamus is shown in Figure 4.3; the brainstem consists of the midbrain, pons, and medulla, as shown in Figure 4.2; and the intermediolateral cell column is shown in the left half of Figure 4.2 as a series of cell bodies arranged vertically within the spinal cord.

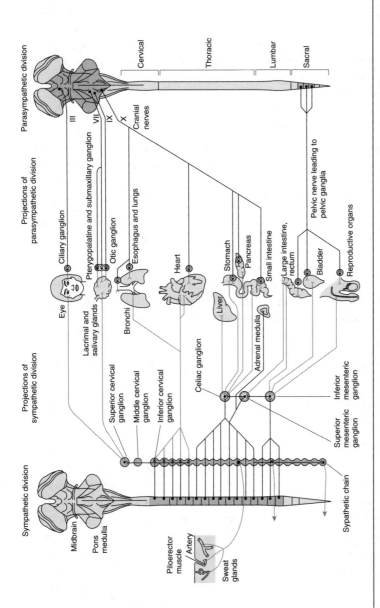

Figure 4.2 The autonomic nervous system. The sympathetic and parasympathetic branches are shown. The enteric division, not shown separately, here, consists of groups of cell bodies and nerve fibers embedded in the walls of the esophagus, stomach, and intestines. Synapses occur at points where nerve fibers arrive at cell bodies, and neuroeffector junctions are points where autonomic postganglionic fibers arrive at target tissues. Redrawn from Iversen, S., Iversen, L., & Saper, C. B. (2000). The autonomic nervous system and the hypothalamus. In E. R. Kandel, J. H. Schwartz & T. M. Jessell (Eds.), *Principles of Neural Science* (4th ed.). New York: McGraw-Hill. Copyright © 2000 by McGraw-Hill. Used with permission.

2. *Ganglia.* Ganglia are collections of cell bodies and their internal connections. The autonomic ganglia constitute the primary way station for autonomic motor signals descending from the spinal cord and for sensory messages returning from the respective organs and tissues. They also are the first stage of integration of these forms of nerve activity. For this reason, the ganglia are part of the local regulatory system that acts in concert with the internal reflexes possessed by each organ. In all ganglia, the primary neurotransmitter is acetylcholine. As part of the local integration of autonomic function, the ganglia also regulate the local traffic to and from their target organs through neuropeptides and neuromodulators. These provide a degree of organ-specific regulation that would otherwise not occur.

3. *Postganglionic fibers.* Postganglionic fibers travel from the autonomic ganglia to their target tissues. Because they are outputs from a ganglion, their messages are not the same as the messages carried by preganglionic fibers. They are more elaborated and refined by locally derived information.

4. *Neuroeffector junctions.* A neuroeffector junction is a point at which postganglionic fibers act to alter the motor function of smooth muscles in the autonomically innervated organs. A neuroeffector junction itself has the character of a synapse between two neurons, but instead the autonomic nerve terminal secretes packets of its particular neurotransmitter on an appropriate receptor that is part of the target tissue. The target cell is either a smooth muscle cell, a cardiac muscle cell, or a secretory endocrine cell. Therefore, a neuroeffector junction is a point where a nerve impulse is translated into a motor action in a local tissue, allowing it to adjust its activity and change the state of the organism's regulation.

The Sympathetic Nervous System

As shown in Figure 4.2, the sympathetic nerves exit from the spinal cord along the thoracic and lumbar regions. They send preganglionic fibers to a series of interconnected ganglia known as the paravertebral chain ganglia. A preganglionic sympathetic fiber may synapse immediately with a postganglionic fiber, which in turn travels to its target organ. Or the preganglionic fiber may travel up or down the chain ganglia before synapsing with one or more postganglionic fibers. In fact, most sympathetic preganglionic fibers do both of these things: They synapse with a postganglionic fiber at one level and send a collateral branch to another level in the chain, synapsing with several other postganglionic fibers along the way. In addition, some sympathetic preganglionics may travel directly to more distant ganglia controlling the actions of the digestive system, the large intestine, the bladder, and the genitalia.

In the sympathetic branch, each preganglionic fiber will synapse with an average of 10 postganglionic fibers. As a result of this 1:10 pre- to postganglionic ratio and the extensive linkages across widely distributed ganglia, the activities of the sympathetic postganglionic fibers tend to be highly coordinated with one another and to act very broadly on target organs. Accordingly, the actions of various target organs tend to be closely integrated. In fact, the sympathetic branch was so named because the concerted nature of its actions causes organs to act in sympathy with one another.

Sympathetic postganglionic fibers control the activity of smooth muscle cells, cardiac muscle cells, or cardiac pacemaker cells by secreting norepinephrine at the neuroeffector junction. The action of norepinephrine is generally to enhance the rate and force of contraction of the smooth muscle and cardiac muscle cells and the rate of discharge of the cardiac pacemakers. Thus, the sympathetic nervous system generally increases the state of activation and function of the organs it supplies.

A notable exception to this description of fiber organization and target tissues occurs in the case of the medulla of the adrenal glands, which are located above the kidneys. Sympathetic nerve fibers to the adrenal gland reach neurosecretory cells, not smooth muscle cells. The adrenal medulla receives sympathetic preganglionic fibers directly from the spinal cord that do not synapse at a sympathetic ganglion. These sympathetic fibers therefore secrete acetylcholine, as do all preganglionics. This cholinergic stimulation causes the adrenal medulla to secrete the catecholamines epinephrine and norepinephrine into the bloodstream, where epinephrine acts as an endocrine messenger.

A second exception to the norepinephrine-secretion rule is seen in the sympathetic innervation of the sweat glands on the soles of our feet and the palms of our hands. The sympathetic nerves secrete acetylcholine at these glands to cause them to produce sweat. These sweat glands are especially sensitive to our emotional state, and the sudden increase in skin moisture when we are nervous is thought to make our hands and feet grip better in response to emergencies.

The sympathetic nervous system is always active during normal homeostasis and becomes more active during times of stress. It plays an essential role in the body's adjustments to normal demands in concert with the parasympathetic nervous system, and it is essential for the integration and expression of the fight-or-flight response during times of stress. The fight-or-flight response is a highly integrated set of cardiovascular and endocrine changes designed to prepare for and support vigorous, even violent, physical activity involved in literally fighting or fleeing for one's life—just the sort of primitive behaviors designed to support survival in a threatening, life-or-death natural environment.

The Parasympathetic Nervous System

The parasympathetic nervous system, again as shown in Figure 4.2, sends fibers to its target organs by way of the cranial nerves arising from the brainstem and by way of the sacral segment of the spinal cord. These fibers travel some distance from the cord to ganglia located close to, or inside of, the target organs. This close proximity of the ganglia to the target tissues is a major anatomical and functional feature distinguishing the parasympathetic system from the sympathetic. Unlike the highly interconnected ganglia of the sympathetic branch, the parasympathetic ganglia are isolated from one another.

In addition to having widely separated ganglia, the parasympathetic nervous system has a small number of preganglionic fibers relative to postganglionic fibers. Each preganglionic fiber gives rise to an average of three postganglionics. This 1:3 ratio and separation of function among the ganglia suggests that activity at parasympathetic target tissues is highly localized and specific to the needs of the separate organs.

The postganglionic parasympathetic fibers all act by secreting acetylcholine onto specialized cholinergic receptors located on smooth muscle fibers or the heart muscle and cardiac pacemakers. In the gut, parasympathetic fibers function to stimulate gastric activity to permit digestion of food. In contrast to the sympathetic division's support of fight-or-flight responses, the parasympathetic division generally supports feeding, energy storage, and reproduction. In the case of most organs, the actions of these two autonomic branches oppose one another, allowing a smoothly graded activity of the target organ.

The Enteric Nervous System

The enteric branch of the autonomic nervous system is the most specialized of the three. As the name implies, it is located entirely near or within the organs of digestion, including the pancreas, the gall bladder, and the gastrointestinal tract. These organs are able to act quite independently of outside control because their intrinsic sensory nerves communicate to sets of interneurons and motor output neurons in enteric ganglia that are able to control the organs in question. Its neurotransmitter is acetylcholine.

Table 4.1   Autonomic Nervous System Effects on Target Organs

Organ	Sympathetic	Parasympathetic
Eye	Pupillary dilation	Pupillary constriction
Saliva glands	Viscous saliva	Watery saliva
Lung	Bronchial dilation	Bronchial constriction
Heart	Increased rate, force	Decreased rate, force
Blood vessels	Constriction	No effect
Intestines	Decreased secretion and peristalsis	Increased secretion and peristalsis
Bladder	Relaxation	Contraction
Adrenal medulla	Epinephrine secretion	No effect

Some consider the enteric system to be a branch of the autonomic nervous system, and some consider it part of the digestive system. The entire enteric system is in turn controlled by the other two branches of the autonomic nervous system.

Coordinated Actions of the Autonomic Branches

Although the autonomic nervous system has three branches and many organs to regulate, some useful generalizations describe its actions and its effects on its target organs. The sympathetic and parasympathetic branches tend to oppose one another so that the joint activation of the branches can allow a graded, reciprocal regulation of organic function. The brainstem nuclei governing the two branches also communicate in such a way that increased activation of one usually signals inhibition of another. This is relatively well understood in the case of the actions of the heart. As Figure 4.2 shows, the heart, like most organs, has dual sympathetic and parasympathetic innervation. Parasympathetic activity lessens the force and rate of contraction of the heart, whereas sympathetic activity increases these functions. In the case of the enteric nervous system, parasympathetic activation tends to increase activity of the organs of digestion, and so it complements the actions of the enteric nervous system. The sympathetic nervous system tends to inhibit actions of the digestive system and so opposes the actions of the enteric nervous system. The enteric nervous system acts primarily on and within the viscera of the digestive tract and consists primarily of local ganglia that receive inputs from a single organ and reflexively regulate the activity of that organ. Table 4.1 summarizes the effects of autonomic activity at major target organs.

Central Autonomic Control by the Brainstem

In discussing homeostatic regulation above the autonomic nervous system, we will refer to the several structures of the central nervous system. These are shown in Figure 4.3 for purposes of orientation.

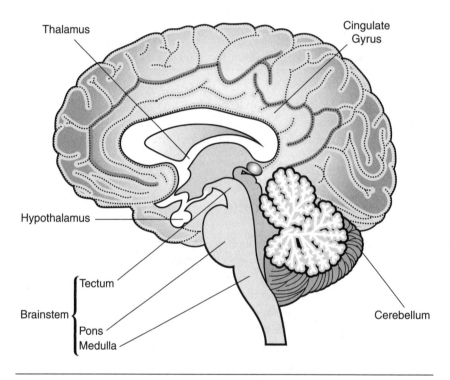

Figure 4.3   The central nervous system, including the cerebral hemisphere, hypothalamus, brainstem, and spinal cord.

Hypothalamic Integration of Autonomic, Endocrine, and Motor Functions

The hypothalamus does three things that place it at the top level of normal homeostatic organization: (a) It provides inputs to the brainstem, thus modifying its autonomic regulation; (b) it controls endocrine function and integrates this with brainstem activity; and (c) it has centers that influence posture and locomotion. The hypothalamus is also in contact with higher brain centers, including structures associated with emotional states and areas such as the frontal cortex. These centers serve conscious decision making, planning, and goal directedness. Therefore, we might characterize the hypothalamus as maintaining the highest level of organization over more basic homeostatic regulation and as being the way station for communication with brain regions that serve still larger goals related to survival.

A dramatic illustration of the ability of the hypothalamus and brainstem to regulate homeostasis, including even relatively complex behaviors, came from classic experiments by Walter Cannon and his colleague Philip Bard (see Bard, 1928). In their quest to understand the organization of the central nervous system, they employed a simple but powerful technique. They asked how well an animal, in this case a cat, could survive and function if different parts of the brain were removed. By systematically cutting the brain at different levels and testing the animals after recovery from the surgery, it became possible to make some broad inferences about the degree of behavioral and homeostatic regulation controlled at different levels of the brain and brainstem. Figure 4.4 shows the brain of a cat with transactions at three different levels of the upper brainstem and hypothalamus. The preparation shown in (a) yielded results that are instructive to our discussion of the hypothalamus but also for the larger purpose of this book. It indicates a cat brain in which the cerebral cortex has been cut just above the level of the hypothalamus. Cats with cuts at this level that spared the cerebellum and brainstem were able to sustain life in the laboratory with little difficulty as long as they were provided with food and water. This showed that all of the homeostatic functions were retained at the level of the hypothalamus and brainstem.

Perhaps more revealing of the brain's organization were the complex behaviors that remained. The cats would right themselves and land on their feet if they were held high and dropped in an awkward posture, showing that their motor systems were intact and able to respond to sensory inputs. More impressively, they would exhibit "sham rage" if even mildly provoked, such as by stroking the fur. The animal assumed a threat posture, hissed, and would attempt to bite and scratch, exhibiting a stereotyped behavioral complex that also had autonomic and endocrine components. As complex as these responses were, they were referred to as sham rage because the response was poorly directed at an outside cause, was stereotyped, and subsided more quickly than would a true rage response in an intact animal. Cuts at the lower levels shown in (b) and (c) resulted in increasingly fragmentary and reflexlike components of these behaviors,

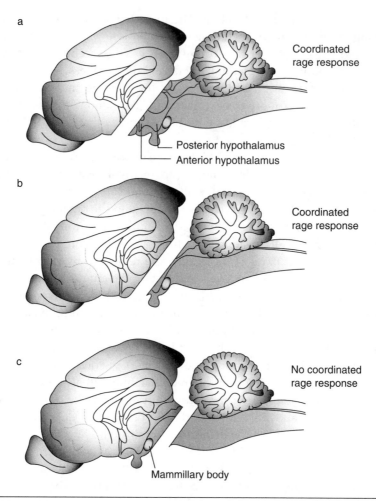

a

Coordinated
rage response

Posterior hypothalamus
Anterior hypothalamus

b

Coordinated
rage response

c

No coordinated
rage response

Mammillary body

Figure 4.4 Cannon and Bard's cat preparation. (a) The cat's cerebral cortex has been removed above the level of the hypothalamus. The cat was able to produce a fully coordinated "sham rage" display to stimuli such as stroking. This sham rage was stereotyped and not focused on a specific target. This preparation demonstrated that the hypothalamus and lower structures had the necessary motor and visceral integrative networks to produce this fully integrated response. (b) The cat's hypothalamus has been cut between its anterior and posterior divisions. Most of the elements of the sham rage were retained, indicating that the posterior hypothalamus retained the essential structures to coordinate behavioral and visceral outputs. (c) The cut has been made below the hypothalamus. The response of the cat to tactile stimuli became fragmented and poorly coordinated, indicating that the visceral and motor components of expression of the emotions were no longer jointly regulated by the hypothalamus.

and the researchers had greater difficulty in keeping the animals alive. This set of experiments illustrated for the first time the degree to which the hypothalamus organized elaborate survival-related behaviors in conjunction with autonomic and endocrine regulation. It also opened up investigations into the neurophysiology of the emotions, a topic we address in Chapters 6 and 7.

Later investigations revealed the hypothalamus to be a collection of specialized groups of nuclei that could be placed in three functional divisions: the endocrine, the autonomic, and the skeletal motor. A detailed discussion of the anatomy and organization of these hypothalamic nuclei is presented in Kandel et al. (2000, ch. 49). Here we focus on the functions of the hypothalamus in relation to stress and emotions more generally.

The primary hypothalamic nucleus that regulates endocrine and autonomic function during stress is the *paraventricular nucleus*. This nucleus is a large, complex group of functionally distinct divisions. These are diagrammed in Figure 4.5a. One of these divisions, the dorsal and ventral parvocellular division, projects to the brainstem and spinal cord, where it can modify autonomic regulation and descending message traffic. The medial parvocellular division has neurosecretory neurons that project to the median eminence of the hypothalamus, the way station to the pituitary gland. As the diagram shows, this nucleus is adjacent to the third ventricle, lying midline in the brain. As shown in Figure 4.5b, cells of the median eminence secrete peptide messengers into the pituitary stalk, where they travel to the anterior pituitary. The posterior pituitary receives hypothalamic secretory nerve fibers directly.

Two stress-related peptides secreted by the hypothalamus are corticotropin releasing factor (CRF) and arginine vasopressin (AVP). AVP (also known as antidiuretic hormone) is released at the posterior pituitary, where it enters the general circulation to regulate excretion of water by the kidneys. At the anterior pituitary, AVP and CRF cause the secretion of ACTH and beta-endorphin by the anterior pituitary. Some neurons of the paraventricular nucleus synthesize CRF only, some AVP only, and some both CRF and AVP. The joint actions of CRF and AVP at the anterior pituitary play a major role in the stress response by greatly enhancing the pituitary's output of ACTH.

The Endocrine Response During Stress

The endocrine response during stress has two parallel arms, the adreno-medullary response, controlled by the sympathetic nervous system, and

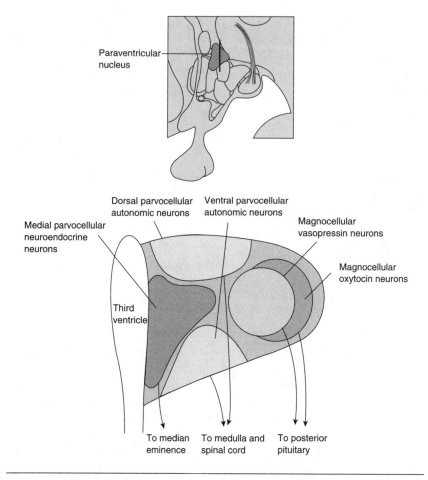

Figure 4.5 The hypothalamus and its paraventricular nucleus. The top figure indicates the location of the hypothalamus and the paraventricular nucleus within it. The lower figure shows that the paraventricular nucleus contains several sub-nuclei. The regulation of cortisol secretion is controlled by neurosecretory cells of the medial parvocellular division. Corticotropin releasing factor (CRF) fibers from this area project to the median eminence, where CRF is released into the portal circulation of the anterior pituitary gland. The dorsal and ventral parvocellular divisions project to the brainstem autonomic nuclei and the spinal cord, where they can alter autonomic outflow.

the adrenocortical response, controlled by the hypothalamus and pituitary. These are diagrammed in Figure 4.6.

During states of stress, the adrenal medulla secretes epinephrine and norepinephrine into the circulation. The adrenal medulla is activated by

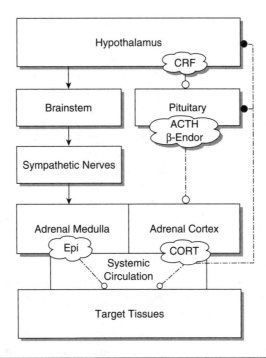

Figure 4.6   Neuroendocrine components of the stress response. Functional organization of the systems controlling release of the primary stress hormones cortisol, beta-endorphine, and epinephrine.

sympathetic preganglionic fibers originating in the brainstem *nucleus of the solitary tract.* These sympathetic outputs are in turn influenced by messages arising from the paraventricular nucleus of the hypothalamus. Epinephrine is an endocrine messenger to many organ systems, where it acts on beta-adrenoreceptors located at points accessible to diffusion from the bloodstream. In general, the action of epinephrine reinforces the actions of the sympathetic nerves. Although norepinephrine also enters the bloodstream from the adrenal gland, its actions on target tissues are negligible. The alpha-adrenoreceptors that are sensitive to norepinehrine have sympathetic nerve endings with tight neuroeffector junctions that are relatively distant from the blood supply, and they are not readily activated by blood-borne norepinephrine. Therefore, norepinephrine has little role as a stress hormone.

The second major stress hormone is cortisol. Unlike epinephrine, cortisol plays a role both in normal states of activity and during periods

Table 4.2   Cortisol Effects on Target Tissues

Tissue	Effect
Neuron	Enhanced catecholamine synthesis
Hippocampus	Enhanced memory function
Thalamus	Sensitivity to incoming stimuli
Adrenoreceptors	Enhanced alpha and receptor sensitivity
Adrenal medulla	Enhanced catecholamine synthesis
Immune system	Enhanced and inhibited
Inflammation	Inhibited
Glucose	Enhanced production
Fatty acid	Enhanced liberation
Kidney	Water diuresis and sodium retention

of stress. Cortisol is required for normal cellular and metabolic function, so much so that experimental animals deprived of their adrenal cortex are difficult to keep alive. Cortisol's presence is necessary for normal autonomic function and hence for all forms of physiological regulation. Humans with Addison's disease, an insufficiency of adrenal function, have poor salt and water balance, low blood pressure, and other forms of autonomic dysfunction. Munck, Guyre, and Holbrook (1984) referred to cortisol's actions during normal periods of function as "permissive" because they allow tissues to carry out their normal functions. A partial list of cortisol's effects is given in Table 4.2.

Cortisol secretion shows a very pronounced diurnal rhythm. Its output reaches a peak before awakening, usually about 6:00 a.m., and its levels drop slowly until about noon, when a small rise occurs during the mid-day meal. Cortisol levels vary over the afternoon hours and then decline to a low point during sleep in the early morning hours. The rhythmic diurnal pattern is considered important for maintaining normal organ regulation, and loss of this rhythm is potentially associated with poor long-term health. Cortisol's diurnal cycle is regulated by hypothalamic pacemaker cells controlling neurons that act on the paraventricular nucleus.

Cortisol is regulated by descending outputs that generate its secretion in concert with negative feedback of cortisol to three areas that decrease its production and release. Figure 4.6 shows the *classical negative feedback model,* under which cortisol is secreted from the adrenal gland and distributed by the systemic circulation, and negative feedback occurs at the pituitary and the hypothalamus. Cortisol reaches the pituitary directly via the bloodstream. It returns to the hypothalamus indirectly by way of the circulation and its contact with cerebrospinal fluid in the ventricles. The proximity of the paraventricular nucleus to the third ventricle is therefore the route of this negative feedback. A final locus of cortisol's negative feedback, not shown in Figure 4.6, is the *hippocampus*. The hippocampus is usually associated with memory formation, but it is now also seen as the primary site of cortisol's negative feedback. When cortisol is absent, tonic inputs from the hippocampus act through neuronal fibers traveling indirectly to the paraventricular nucleus of the hypothalamus, causing it to stimulate CRF secretion. When cortisol levels are high, this tonic activity of the hippocampus is regulated by negative feedback of cortisol acting on specialized hippocampal receptors.

Cortisol also participates in the stress response. Without cortisol's tonic influences on normal function, the stress apparatus would not be in proper condition to respond to emergencies. Cortisol is necessary for the normal synthesis and function of both alpha- and beta-adrenoreceptors. In its absence, the actions of the autonomic nerves would be greatly diminished, and epinephrine would be less effective at its target tissues. Stress levels of cortisol potentiate activities of the sympathetic nervous system to increase the release of stored glucose and fats. These metabolic functions help provide fuel substrates to support fight-or-flight reactions. Munck et al. (1984) characterized cortisol's acute actions during periods of stress as *regulatory:* that is, exerting *negative feedback* at the level of the central nervous system and controlling the stress response itself. In the absence of cortisol, stress responses have damaging effects. Munck and his colleagues viewed cortisol during acute stress responses as preventing the stress response itself from threatening the individual's homeostasis. This important regulatory action is seen in experimental animals whose adrenal glands are removed. In addition to being impaired in their normal metabolic functions, adrenalectomized animals frequently die during periods of stress due to poor regulation of the stress response. The actions of cortisol during stress and its regulatory role will be discussed in more detail in Chapter 7.

Cortisol and epinephrine can integrate widespread functions due to their ability to reach all tissues via the systemic circulation and thereby to significantly alter the background environment in which those tissues operate. In addition to the integration of organic function achieved by the opposing dual effects of sympathetic and parasympathetic fibers, simultaneous endocrine influences modulate and coordinate activity and responses across many tissues.

A third stress hormone is beta-endorphin. In response to CRF from the hypothalamus, the pituitary produces equal quantities of beta-endorphin and ACTH. Beta-endorphin is a potent agonist of opiate receptors in the nervous system, producing analgesia, among other effects. Because beta-endorphin is released along with ACTH and cortisol during stress, it appears to act as an analgesic in preparation for potential pain or injury and possibly to regulate moods during such times.

Summary

A survey of control over organic function, starting with the intrinsic controls by the organs and moving up through the autonomic nervous system, brainstem, and hypothalamus, shows that the vital functions of the body are functionally autonomous, with regulation and integrated controls being applied in a layered fashion as we move up the system. This hierarchical control scheme is designed to coordinate the activities of otherwise isolated tissues and organs and organize their function in increasingly concerted ways so that their integrated actions may serve higher survival purposes. Although these controls need no voluntary control to operate properly, they are subject to intervention by higher control centers. In terms of our larger agenda to describe how psychological stress influences the actions of the body—or, as we said before, to answer the question of how an idea can change the body—we will later describe the modification of these autonomic and endocrine activities by the higher brain centers comprised by the cortex and limbic system. These intervening controls will be emphasized in Chapter 6's discussion of higher mental and emotional functions that act on this organizational scheme from the top down.

Further Reading

Bear, M. F., Connors, B. W., & Paradiso, M. A. (2001). *Neuroscience: Exploring the brain* (2nd ed.). Baltimore: Lippincott, Williams, & Wilkins.

A basic neurosciences text with excellent neuroanatomical illustrations. An excellent overview of some aspects of endocrine and autonomic function is given in Chapter 18.

Cannon, W. B. (1935). Stresses and strains of homeostasis (Mary Scott Newbold Lecture). *American Journal of Medical Sciences, 189,* 1–14.

A basic statement of Cannon's views on homeostasis.

Kandel, E. R., Schwartz, J. H., & Jessell, T. M. (2000). *Principles of neuroscience* (4th ed.). New York: McGraw-Hill.

A fundamental textbook of the neurosciences with a strong blending of neuroanatomy, physiology, and behavior. Chapter 49 is an excellent overview of the autonomic nervous system and hypothalamus that provides a detailed discussion of these parts of the nervous system. Chapter 50 reviews the neural basis of the emotions, an essential basis for understanding the stress response.

5

Physical and Psychological Stress

To consider the possible effects of long-term stress on the body, we should first examine the acute changes that occur during brief periods of stress. This information helps answer our original question about how ideas can have power over the body and how stress mechanisms can affect disease processes. To do so, we will consider stress reactions that originate from physical causes or that begin as psychological responses.

We might ask what reason there is to distinguish between psychological and physical stress. Because of our interest in psychological aspects of stress, we examine these representative stressors in terms of the top-down versus bottom-up nature of their activational properties. At one extreme is physical exercise, which produces pronounced cardiovascular and endocrine responses primarily because the physical demands of the working muscles and respiratory system send ascending signals to the brain, a *bottom-up* patterning of activation. At the other extreme is mental arithmetic, which involves *top-down* activation due to intense mental effort to perform arithmetic calculations in working memory. Its ability to activate cardiovascular control centers in the brainstem is therefore related to signals from higher centers. The top-down organization of such stressors provides us with the beginnings of a working model of psychological stress.

We will also consider each stressor in terms of its *activating* and *appetitive-aversive* qualities. The total physiological response to a behavioral challenge results from activation associated with the demands of the situation and the emotions it evokes. Challenges that create states of distress associated with negative emotions differentially result in cortisol secretion.

Although physical and psychological stressors may have similar acute effects on the body, an important characteristic of psychological stressors is that they may not have clear onsets and offsets. We carry them around with us, so to speak, and they account for most of what people commonly refer to as stress in their lives. Developing a useful way of thinking about the mechanisms of psychological stress is therefore a central theme of this book.

Classes of Stress Responses

There are several schemes for classifying stressors. Here we consider physical versus psychological stressors and view their effects in terms of activation and appetitive-aversive qualities. There are also several schemes for classifying stress reactions. Studies of stress in animals have yielded two major patterns of reaction to stressor challenge. The first concerns cases of *threat to control*, in which the organism is actively striving to maintain or gain control over the environment. Threat to control evokes either an immediate assertion of control over the situation or an effortful attempt to gain control. The physiological response during such active efforts to control the environment is known as the *defense reaction*. The examples of exercise and the fight-or-flight response discussed in this chapter both fall into this category. However, the emotions involved may differ between the two. The second pattern concerns situations of actual *loss of control* over the environment. This has been termed the *defeat reaction*, and it has relevance for understanding the effects of *failure to control* in studies on humans. In Chapter 8, we will consider the effects of loss of control and the resulting experience of helplessness on persons and animals. A short review of this classification scheme and some major components of the physiological responses during each situation are provided by Folkow (1993).

The animal literature contains a significant number of studies comparing defense reactions with defeat reactions. Many of these studies involve aggressive encounters between two members of the species and an examination of the physiological responses of the winner and loser of these encounters. The exact responses in each case are complex because there exists for each species a unique set of social relations determining all aspects of the behavioral interaction between individuals. For example, chimpanzees, which live in social groups, have very different rules for determining dominance and the nature of aggressive encounters than do orangutans, which are more solitary and less likely to have aggressive encounters. Similarly, leaf-eating monkeys have different levels of activity and aggression than do fruit-eating monkeys. Factors such as social conditions and food type interact with a historically determined set of relationships between individuals and their conspecific aggressors and natural predators. These well-developed interactions have a family of related endocrine and physiological adjustments that differ somewhat across species, as noted by Weiner (1992, ch. 7). In this chapter, we compare exercise and fight-or-flight reactions as two varieties of defense reaction.

We are also making a different kind of distinction in this chapter, between psychological and physiological or physical stressors: that is, stressors that start out in the body and ones that start out as ideas, fears, and sources of anxiety and only later become part of the workings of the body. We should keep in mind that these sources of stress arising in a fully conscious person or animal are not completely separable: Awareness will intrude on most situations, and with awareness comes a view toward future consequences, often a source of psychological stress.

The Exercise Response

Exercise has two major components: the *preparatory* phase and the *active* phase. During exercise, substantial changes occur in cardiovascular activity and hormonal output. The purpose of these adjustments is to provide maximum oxygen and fuel to the exercising muscles. An excellent review of the exercise response can be found in Smith, Guyton, Manning, and White (1976). A brief overview of cardiovascular function may be found in Rushmer (1989), and more detail may be found in Guyton and Hall (2000).

The Preparatory Phase

Physiologists have noted that humans and animals preparing for exercise often show dramatic changes in physiological function before the start of any significant muscular activity. This has led to the recognition that centrally generated commands from the cortex can result in altered hypothalamic and brainstem functions controlling autonomic outflow (Hobbs, 1982). These preparatory changes mimic those during exercise. For example, in trained runners preparing to start an actual race, resting heart rates were found to double as the starter was calling out the starting commands (McArdle, Foglia, & Patti, 1967). The rise in heart rate was greatest in sprinters starting a 60-yard dash (67 to 148 beats per minute), smaller in preparation for a 220-yard dash (67 to 130 beats per minute), and still less in middle-distance runners starting an 880-yard run (62 to 122 beats per minute).

Evidence from animal studies shows that the preparatory phase is initiated in the prefrontal cortex, suggesting activation of a planned, intentional set of preparatory changes. Activity in the prefrontal cortex then gives rise to increased activity of the supplementary motor cortex, the premotor cortex, and the primary motor cortex.

These cortical changes result in descending influences that activate the hypothalamus and brainstem nuclei associated with sympathetic activation and suppression of parasympathetic activity. These top-down processes result in increased heart rate, increased cardiac output, increased sympathetic outflow to the blood vessels, and increased epinephrine secretion. There is some uncertainty about the amount of vasoconstriction of the blood vessels accompanying preparation for exercise. It is likely that some combination of circulating epinephrine and autonomically mediated changes causes dilation of some muscle vascular beds, resulting in increased muscle blood flow. The net effect of these changes is an increase in blood pressure, with a proportionally greater rise in systolic pressure than diastolic pressure. The top-down nature of these cortical influences is illustrated by the active inhibition of the baroreceptor reflex by cortical influences, as described in Chapter 4.

We will return to a discussion of the preparatory phase after describing the changes actually occurring during exercise. These anticipatory changes will provide a basis for thinking about mental stress and its effects on the body.

The Active Phase

During the initiation of exercise, muscular work commences, with the result that the descending cerebral influences referred to in the preparatory phase are now enhanced by (a) neural feedback from muscular contraction, (b) peripherally induced changes in blood vessel function, and (c) return of blood to the heart. The combination of muscle contraction, vascular dilation, and increased sympathetic function results in very significant increases in cardiac output, amounting to as much as six times that of resting levels. As a result, cardiac output may rise from about 4 L/min in a resting adult man to 24 L/min at maximum exercise (Smith et al., 1976). The changes in cardiac output during exercise result from a combination of centrally induced motor commands, acting on autonomic centers, and feedback from the periphery, but the larger influence is the peripheral one.

Peripheral Blood Flow in Exercise

Sympathetic outflow to all the blood vessels increases substantially during exercise. As a result, blood flow in nonworking muscles does not change appreciably from resting values, and blood flow to the viscera actually decreases. This generalized increase in vascular tonus also results in increased tension on the walls of the large veins that conduct blood back to the heart, thereby improving the return of blood to the heart. However, in spite of increased sympathetically mediated constriction of the blood vessels in nonworking muscles and the viscera, local mechanisms ensure that an adequate supply of blood reaches the working muscles. The exercising muscles produce metabolites due to their increased use of oxygen and fuel. These metabolites result in relaxation of the muscle layer of the resistance vessels of the working muscles, causing substantial increases in blood flow, which may reach eight times that of resting levels.

The combination of descending autonomic influences and local metabolic influences results in a redistribution of blood flow, allowing significant increases of oxygen and nutrients to reach the exercising muscles. As a result of these increases, a trained runner may maintain 85% of maximum effort for periods of 3 to 5 hours.

Cardiac Output During Exercise

The other major component of the cardiovascular adjustment to exercise involves profound changes in the activity of the heart. First, the improved return of blood to the heart results in better filling of the left ventricle during the brief period of relaxation prior to each beat. This improved filling results in greater stretch of the muscular wall of the atria and ventricles. It is a basic property of cardiac muscle to contract more effectively in response to increased stretch, a response known as the Frank-Starling reflex. Therefore, the redistribution of blood volume and flow caused by sympathetic output and increased muscle metabolism results in improvement of the pumping action of the heart because of the intrinsic Frank-Starling mechanism. This results in an increased *stroke volume*, the amount of blood the heart expels on each beat.

Second, during exercise, the increase in feedback from exercising muscle to the brainstem cardiovascular control centers results in a suppression of parasympathetic activity and an increase in sympathetic outflow from the brainstem cardiovascular control centers. This shift to a dominant sympathetic pattern of outflow results in a substantial increase in heart rate. Highly trained athletes may have resting heart rates of 35 to

40 beats per minute, whereas during exercise they may maintain sustained rates of 180 beats per minute, indicating a four- to fivefold increase.

Third, the contractile force of the heart may increase during exercise. This results from (a) increased sympathetic outflow to the heart, acting to improve contractile force of the left ventricle, and (b) the increase in circulating epinephrine, which augments this improved contractility by acting on beta-adrenergic receptors on cardiac muscle.

We therefore see three influences acting in concert to improve the action of the heart as a pump: improved filling of the left ventricle, increased frequency of contraction, and increased force of contraction. These lead to increased cardiac output and increased blood flow to the working muscles.

Endocrine Changes During Exercise

The changes in cardiovascular activity during exercise are accompanied by supporting changes in endocrine function. Endocrine responses enhance cardiovascular function directly and support muscular work by increasing the availability of fuel.

Epinephrine, secreted by the adrenal medulla, acts to augment autonomically mediated changes in the heart and blood vessels. First, epinephrine increases cardiac contractility. Second, it increases dilation of blood vessels in exercising muscles by acting on beta-adrenoreceptors in the blood vessel wall. This works to decrease vascular resistance in exercising muscles, augmenting the metabolic dilation mentioned above. Third, epinephrine increases the liberation of stored fat, allowing free fatty acids to enter the circulation and travel to exercising muscles for utilization as fuel.

Cortisol, secreted by the cortex of the adrenal gland located above the kidney, is critical for the liberation of stored glucose and fat. Sometime after the onset of exercise, the increased use of circulating glucose as fuel for the muscles will result in a drop in blood glucose levels. This is a signal to the hypothalamus and pituitary to increase the release of ACTH to signal increased production of cortisol. Cortisol then increases the liberation into the bloodstream of glucose from the liver and free fatty acids from adipose tissues.

Beta-endorphin is secreted by the pituitary in equal amounts along with ACTH. Beta-endorphin is known to be an opiate analogue and to activate brain receptor sites associated with opioid analgesia. It may also have mood-elevating effects. This system is thought to modulate the discomfort associated with severe muscle effort and to modulate moods during fight-or-flight situations.

Exercise and Adaptation to Stress

Selye recognized that exposure to a stressor could increase the body's ability to cope with that stressor in the future by a process of physiological adaptation. Exercise is an excellent example of increased coping with repeated exposure. Physical training involves doing a set of exercises with increasing intensity over an extended period. The increase in ability with training is an example of adaptation to the required effort.

Selye also noted that severe and extended exposure to any stressor could ultimately exceed the ability of the system to cope or adapt. Similarly, it is possible for a person who enjoys exercise to increase the level of physical demand from session to session beyond the body's ability to respond adaptively and recover fully, making the exercise a source of long-term physical stress. Runners habitually training more than 45 miles per week at moderate to high intensity are known to have chronically elevated cortisol levels and negative mood states (Luger et al., 1987). Too much physical training can produce a state of overtraining that may take months of abstinence from exercise for full recovery. The overtraining phenomenon appears to illustrate how a protracted allostatic load can exert a deleterious effect on the person's well-being.

The Fight-or-Flight Response

As Claude Bernard postulated, all living systems must have methods of self-protection, whether that means compensating for minor variations in the temperature, fighting off invading organisms, or fleeing a predator. As organisms became more complex, so did the repertoire of responses to fend off harm. It seems reasonable that organisms better equipped to defend themselves would have a survival and evolutionary advantage over those less equipped. In higher organisms, there appears to be a general adaptive advantage to those who can flee most effectively from danger or fight off a potential rival or aggressor. Physiologists and psychologists use the generic term *fight-or-flight response* in reference to this loosely defined constellation of functions.

We consider the fight-or-flight response a prototype stress response. It is an energetically intense set of behavioral and physiological changes, undertaken in the interest of maintaining life in the most acutely threatening circumstances. The fight-or-flight response incorporates powerful emotional components and equally powerful exercise-related neuroendocrine and physiological changes.

The *emotions* associated with fight-or-flight are ones we normally consider unpleasant or negative. These include (a) *anxiety,* a sense of apprehension and the anticipation of harm even in the absence of an immediate threat; (b) *fear,* an aroused state felt in the presence of the threat itself; and (c) *anger,* an outwardly directed destructive impulse. These separable but overlapping emotions, accompanied by neuroendocrine and physiological reactions, motivate adaptive behaviors during threatening circumstances. A primary characteristic of all fight-or-flight situations is that the organism has limited control over the outcome. Therefore, it is not certain at the outset that serious injury or death can be avoided. In fact, capture and the helplessness associated with forced immobility are known to be among the most profound of aversive stressors. Tonic immobilization of an experimental animal is therefore used as a highly reproducible and useful laboratory stressor.

The *endocrine changes* associated with the emotions during fight or flight are generally those that increase the vigor and strength of overt behavior, intensify the physiological reactions, and assist in liberating energy stores to enhance the likelihood of successful flight or self-defense. Endocrine substances are transported by the blood and are able to integrate widespread elements of complex responses. The primary hormones underlying the fight-or-flight response are cortisol, beta-endorphin, and epinephrine.

The *autonomic nervous system* changes associated with the fight-or-flight response are a general suppression of parasympathetic activity and increased sympathetic activity. This implies a shift from the energy-storing and conserving functions served by the parasympathetic branch to energy-expending functions associated with gross muscular activity and physical effort necessary to flee from or struggle with an opponent. These changes are the same as would occur during exercise, and the information on autonomic changes during exercise may be applied equally well here.

The fight-or-flight response can be divided into preparatory and active phases similar to the two phases of the exercise response. Anderson and Tosheff (1973) modeled the preparatory and active phases of an aversive encounter by exposing dogs to an active avoidance procedure (active phase) versus having the dogs wait for a prolonged period in the apparatus before the avoidance (preparation phase). The avoidance period was characterized by elevated blood pressure along with increased cardiac output and decreased peripheral resistance, an exerciselike pattern. During preparation, the blood pressure was elevated primarily by increased vascular resistance with a small decrease in cardiac output. These phases clearly parallel the active and preparation phases of exercise described above, although the preavoidance period appears to be characterized by higher levels of peripheral resistance than exercise preparation.

For our purposes, the active portion of the fight-or-flight response involves vigorous exercise accompanied by negative emotions and significant elevation of cortisol, beta-endorphin, and epinephrine.

Different Emotions and Motivations Accompany Exercise and Fight-or-Flight

The exercise response in both the preparatory and active phases indicates that the body is capable of substantial adjustments to the demands of vigorous activity. We may think of the exercise response as forming the core of the fight-or-flight response. However, there is a crucial difference between exercise, particularly for enjoyment, and fight-or-flight situations in the motivational state and the emotions accompanying each activity.

Most people choose to exercise for positive reasons. They run, swim, or compete for enjoyment and improved health. The exercising person may feel significant *positive emotions,* along with a feeling of freedom and an intense sense of satisfaction. Such exercise is voluntary, and the person has almost complete *control* over its duration and intensity. The *outcomes,* short of accidental injury, carry significant benefits and few costs. Prolonged strenuous exercise may also produce a metabolically induced secretion of ACTH accompanied by beta-endorphin secretion. The mood alterations associated with beta-endorphin are often referred to as a runner's high. Therefore, exercise may produce largely positive moods, and the associated endocrine changes are primarily a result of demands for fuel by the muscles.

In the case of the fight-or-flight response, we have an organism fleeing or fighting for its existence. The attendant emotions, such as anxiety, fear, and anger, are powerful negative ones. The behavioral outcome of such an encounter is uncertain, and the costs of failure are disastrous. Such situations produce an immediate and substantial elevation of ACTH, beta-endorphin, and cortisol. In contrast, during exercise, the changes in these hormones are induced by the elevated energy demands and are confined to feedback mechanisms at the hypothalamus and pituitary. The changes occurring during fight-or-flight involve descending activation via the frontal cortex and emotion centers in the limbic system, especially the amygdala and septohippocampal complex. In Chapter 8, we will review studies in humans and animals showing the effects of uncertainty in the face of aversive events. We will also discuss research showing profound behavioral, physiological, and neurochemical alterations in animals following prolonged exposure to uncontrollable aversive stimuli such as electric shock. These studies tell us that significant emotionally determined secretion of stress hormones may occur due to loss of control over the environment, the high cost of failure, and negative emotions.

Why Is Exercise Considered Good if It Is a Stressor?

Because stress is usually portrayed as undesirable, it is natural to question why exercise is so often prescribed as beneficial for health and mood enhancement. The answer lies in the motivations and emotions involved in the situation. Exercise is a physical challenge, undertaken in graded doses and allowing the person complete control over the outcome. As long as the person avoids overtraining, exercise may increase physical fitness and often improves mood. This degree of control and the differences in the accompanying emotions make exercise very different from true fight-or-flight situations.

Thus, the impact of a stressor depends heavily on the way the person interprets the situation. Two challenges that are equally physically demanding can have different consequences for the individual based on the interpretation of the situation and the accompanying emotions. Mason (1968, 1975a, 1975b) performed an extensive series of laboratory studies of adaptive mechanisms and stress responses in primates. One of his most pervasive findings was that his monkeys produced high levels of cortisol when exposed to novel challenges in the laboratory but that this response disappeared when the situation became familiar. Mason concluded that the novelty of each situation was a major determinant of its stressor value, suggesting that the psychological reaction to the situation was as important as, or more important than, the event itself.

Psychological Stress

The most obvious sources of threat to the integrity of the organism are the kinds of physical stressors that Selye was mainly concerned with: cold, heat, infection, hemorrhage, and the like. We refer to these as *physical stressors* because they are threats based on their physical ability to cause harm or destroy life. Psychologists and other students of behavior are more often interested in *psychological stressors*. By these we mean challenges that can alter the workings of the body, and perhaps affect health, because of their meaning to the person and the impact of their meaning for the person's daily life, with some awareness of immediate or long-term consequences. Psychological stressors include such events as loss of a loved one, failure to achieve a highly valued goal in life, or a turn for the worse in a significant relationship. These can be acute, traumatic events or long-lasting strains. These things sooner or later happen to everyone, and we accept them as part of the challenge of life, but our task here is to explore how they act on us and what the mediating mechanisms are likely to be. Clearly, such challenges do not pose a threat because they are physically harmful in the way that cold is, so we should consider what mechanism allows a piece of bad news to bring on a crushing sense of oppression, perhaps tears and sorrow, a loss of faith in the future, a sense of hopelessness, and ultimately even illness.

As a start, we turn to the example of anticipation of exercise. The cardiovascular responses occurring in anticipation of exercise are interesting because they suggest that widespread changes can occur in peripheral function exclusively because of changes in brain activity associated with thinking about and preparing for movement. Orville Smith et al. (1993) have provided impressive data from baboons that were living in social groups and were instrumented to provide real-time readouts of physiological activity along with detailed videotaped records of their behavior. These records showed substantial rises in heart rate and blood pressure in monkeys sitting completely still—just before attacking another monkey. As in the preparation for exercise, these cardiovascular changes seem to illustrate the power of the descending influences of an evolving plan of attack, including the presumed experience of emotions like anger or hostility, to significantly alter the state of the body.

The mental arithmetic task, used by Brod (1963) in a series of influential studies of hypertensives, is a prototypical mental stressor. It is really a family of tasks that all require the volunteer to calculate answers to arithmetic problems without paper and pencil and to provide accurate answers as a check on performance. One example is to give the subject a three-digit number and ask him or her to add the digits together and then add the sum to the original number. The answer is yet another three-digit number, and the same calculations are repeated on each new number until the end of the task period. All versions of the task require the subject to devote significant processing resources to working memory. This is an effortful process that can be mildly unpleasant after the first few seconds. The characteristics of the task can be readily manipulated to increase the difficulty of the calculations and the error rates and to alter its positive or negative emotional valence.

Mental arithmetic produces significant decreases in vagal tone to the heart and increases in sympathetically mediated cardiac activity (Hedman, Hjemdahl, Nordlander, & Åström, 1990). This results in significant increases in heart rate and contractility. Vascular resistance is unchanged or slightly increased from baseline (Allen, Obrist, Sherwood, & Crowell, 1987). These cardiovascular changes are primarily due to the mental effort involved, although blood pressure responses are enhanced by the effect of speaking the answers aloud (Linden, 1991). The task is perceived as mildly aversive (al'Absi, Lovallo, McKey, & Pincomb, 1994), and it produces significant increases in cortisol secretion into the bloodstream (al'Absi et al., 1994; Williams et al., 1982). We can therefore think of the mental arithmetic task as a prototype psychological stressor. It produces significant cardiovascular activation, along with a mild sense of aversion and secretion of cortisol. It does these things in the face of minimal motor demands and maximal mental effort. So its ability to alter physiological function, to have an impact on the workings on the body, derives almost exclusively from the activation of brain centers capable of affecting the brainstem and hypothalamic-pituitary axis. These areas will be discussed in detail in Chapters 6 and 7.

Responses to Aversive and Nonaversive Challenges

We have noted that mental arithmetic is perceived as mildly aversive and that it results in increased cortisol secretion. Activational states that carry a strong negative emotional charge will be a frequent point of discussion throughout the rest of this book, and it may be useful to review specific evidence of a connection between negative affect per se and emotionally induced cortisol secretion. To illustrate the importance of accounting for the emotional response to a challenge, we will present in detail two companion studies done in our laboratory that called upon human volunteers to perform tasks with nearly identical physical requirements but substantial differences in their psychological components (Lovallo, Pincomb, & Wilson, 1986b; Lovallo et al., 1985).

In the first study, we were interested in knowing how human volunteers would react to aversive stimuli when trying to control their occurrence under conditions of maximum uncertainty (Lovallo et al., 1985). We could think of the aversive character and lack of control in this experiment as evoking the *psychological components* of the fight-or-flight response. In the second study, the subjects performed a nearly identical task, but this time they could earn money for good performance, and there were no aversive penalties (Lovallo et al., 1986b). We may look at this task in terms of an *activational state* of working for a positive outcome, with little chance of a negative outcome. The psychological difference between these two tasks parallels the psychological difference between exercise, as a positive challenge, and fight-or-flight, as a fear-ridden and uncertain struggle.

Exposure to Noise and Shock

In the first study, young adult men were asked to perform a simple psychomotor task to avoid the presentation of two aversive stimuli, noise and electric shock. The shocks were brief, mild ones known to be safe and harmless. Nevertheless, even mild electric shock feels unpleasant. The noise was brief enough to permit safe levels of exposure but intense enough to produce a strong degree of startle. The psychomotor task was a 15-minute, simple, variable-interval reaction-time task in which the subjects pressed a response key whenever a red light in front of them came on. There were 24 trials, ranging from 4 to 90 seconds between respond signals, and these signals occurred without warning. In addition, the subject was uncertain when a response would be called for and when a response would be fast enough to avoid an unpleasant outcome. Although the subjects were told that if they responded rapidly enough they would avoid receiving an electric shock or noise burst, in fact these were preprogrammed to occur unpredictably on 50% of the trials (four shocks and eight noise bursts). The subjects were also told that if they responded slowly, they *might or might not* receive a shock or noise burst. This prevented the subjects from testing the relationship between reaction time and aversive stimulation. So from the subject's point of view this task involved anxiety, fear, and maximum uncertainty about the timing and exact source of an aversive event. At the same time, in an attempt to avoid unpleasant outcomes, the subject had to maintain continuous attention for the full 15 minutes, to be prepared to react as rapidly as possible at any moment, and to make rapid motor responses to the red lights.

This attempt to cope with the aversive challenge produced changes very much like those in our model of a fight-or-flight response. The subjects experienced the task as *activating* (they reported increased concentration, effort, interest, and tenseness), as would be expected where effort was being expended to control events, and *distressing* (they reported less control and pleasantness and more distress, impatience, and irritation), as would be normal for exposure to aversive stimuli. The cardiovascular pattern, presented in Figure 5.1a, showed increased systolic and diastolic blood pressure. The hemodynamic adjustments underlying this blood pressure rise showed a drop in vascular resistance and an increase in all components of cardiac performance, including increased heart rate and cardiac output, and increased contractile indices, including a rise in Heather's index of contractility and a shortened preejection period. This pattern of subjective and cardiovascular changes was accompanied by significant alterations in neuroendocrine function, as shown in Figure 5.2. Norepinephrine levels in the blood increased significantly, indicating enhanced global sympathetic function. Cortisol levels also increased significantly. We found that baseline cortisol was significantly correlated with reports of distress and that poststress cortisol was related to distress, tension, and irritability.

It should be emphasized that the subjects were sitting still in a recliner chair with their legs elevated for the entire study. The rises in norepinephrine and cortisol suggest a centrally mediated set of responses related to negative emotions and preparation for a fight-or-flight response without any elevated energy expenditure.

Work to Earn Monetary Reward

In our second study, we challenged the subjects with a rewarding, nonaversive version of the same reaction-time task. The major difference was that instead of a threat of noise or shock as a motivator, we paid subjects a 50-cent bonus for each very rapid response (less than 270 msec) they could perform. The behavioral requirements were the same as for the aversive task. Subjects had to maintain extreme alertness to detect the onset of a respond light, they had to be at a heightened state of preparedness, and they had to make rapid button presses to earn rewards.

The results, in Figure 5.1(b), showed the same pattern of cardiovascular change as did the aversive task: Blood pressure was elevated, and vascular resistance showed a slight decline, whereas all indices of cardiac function were in the direction of elevated activation. As in the aversive task, norepinephrine increased significantly from baseline, again indicating globally enhanced sympathetic activation. This pattern of cardiovascular and catecholamine change was similar to that of preparation for exercise. However, the results differed in one important respect. We saw no change in cortisol secretion from baseline to the reward incentive, as shown in Figure 5.2. Subjective reports showed that the task was primarily activating and nonaversive, as we expected.

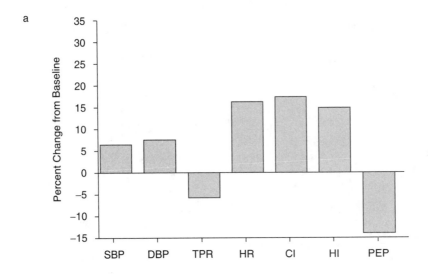

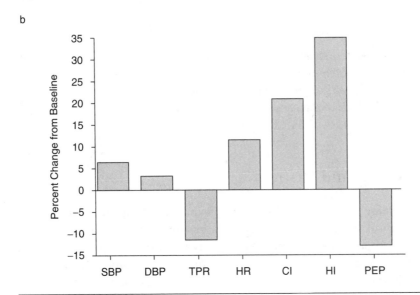

Figure 5.1 Cardiovascular responses during a reaction-time task calling for sustained attention and preparation to carry out rapid motor responses: (a) Reaction-time task using electric shock and loud noise as incentives. (b) Reaction-time task using monetary bonuses as incentives. SBP = systolic blood pressure, DBP = diastolic blood pressure, TPR = total peripheral resistance, HR = heart rate, CI = cardiac index, HI = Heather's index of contractility, PEP = preejection period. (Redrawn From Lovallo et al., 1986 a and b)

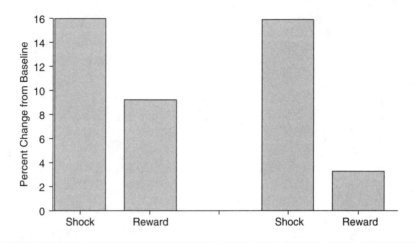

Figure 5.2   Neuroendocrine responses to reaction-time tasks having electric shock or monetary incentives. Left bars indicate norepinephrine responses to shock versus reward. Right bars indicate cortisol responses to these incentives. (Redrawn from Lovallo et al., 1990)

We interpreted these results as showing that activation of attentional and motor response centers in the brain can lead to substantial activation of cardiovascular function even in the absence of significant muscular activity. The lack of increase in cortisol we interpreted as being due to the nonaversive nature of the task.

Activation and Distress

The cardiovascular activation patterns in our examples are similar to the patterns occurring during preparation for exercise and for fight-or-flight. Both tasks required significant mental effort, including heightened attention, and preparation for the execution of a motor plan, resulting in activation of motor areas of the cortex. These behavioral requirements presumably generate strong central commands that engage lower autonomic control centers, resulting in exerciselike cardiovascular adjustments even in the absence of actual exercise.

The strong similarities between the cardiovascular patterns in the two studies indicate that these were associated with the mental effort expended and the similar response requirements of both tasks. Both tasks evoked self-reports of significant concentration, effort, and activation, suggesting that the subjects were actively engaged in the effort of performing as well as possible regardless of the nature of the incentives. This effortful aspect of the tasks therefore seems most closely tied to the cardiovascular changes.

Cortisol responses, in contrast, were different in the two studies. Cortisol increased during the aversive task in relation to its perceived aversiveness, but it did not change in the rewarded task, as shown in Figure 5.2. This suggests that cortisol rises are evoked preferentially by feelings of distress associated with aversive circumstances and are not tied to expenditure of mental effort or to the specific behavioral demands of the tasks. For this reason, we have likened the response to the rewarded task to an exercise preparation response, and we have compared the response to the aversive task to a fight-or-flight response.

Discussion

Substantial changes can occur in peripheral physiology because of mental activity. Preparation for physical exercise, or performing a psychomotor task in the laboratory, can invoke activational changes in cardiovascular function. These changes can occur regardless of the positive or negative emotions involved. They can occur whether the situation is one of fight-or-flight, repeated failures in a contest, or an enjoyable video game.

The cardiovascular response pattern documented for the reaction-time task is not necessarily the same as the pattern seen for other mental stressors. For example, mental arithmetic produces increased heart rate and cardiac output elevations, but it does not result in the same reduction in peripheral resistance that we saw for reaction time (Allen et al., 1987). We suspect that this difference between the tasks in peripheral blood flow regulation has to do with differences in their behavioral requirements. Mental arithmetic primarily engages working memory and does not involve intense preparation for motor activity, although the responses are usually spoken aloud. We may say, therefore, that the pattern of cardiovascular adjustment seen during a mentally challenging task depends on the degree of activation or mental effort the person exerts and on the behavioral characteristics of the task itself.

The emotional component of a task can determine the pattern of endocrine changes, especially the cortisol response. Cortisol can show a prompt and substantial increase in the bloodstream following the onset of potent aversive events such as electric shock. We have noted that the amount of cortisol rise is positively correlated with the negative perceptions of the subjects being tested. This distinction between positive and negative and negative emotional components to a stressor defines what we may think of as states of stress in general and states of *distress* in particular. Stresses placed on the body, either from bottom-up or top-down sources, can be very different in character depending on whether they are neutral to positive in nature or associated with negative affect. We will discuss the consequences of negative affective states, especially the effects of high levels of cortisol in the central nervous system, when we discuss long-term emotional distress in Chapter 7 and the effect of positive affective states on the brain in Chapter 10.

Thus, not all increases in physiological activity from the resting level are signs of distress, and not all such increases signal unhealthy processes. Sometimes these changes are signs of activation in the absence of negative emotions. This distinction between activating and distressing events may be useful for thinking about the influence of mental stress on disease. First, exercise is a health-promoting, beneficial activity accompanied by positive emotional states. Second, the evocation of fight-or-flight responses in nature may differ from the evocation of these primitive reflexes in contemporary life. Charvat, Dell, and Folkow (1964) discussed possible differences in physiological changes associated with normal fight-or-flight reactions that develop rapidly, involve release in exercise, and are terminated when the encounter ends. In modern social settings, where aggressive impulses are inhibited and hostile encounters rarely occur, fight-or-flight reactions may involve prolonged emotional and preparatory changes with no behavioral release. These writers argued that prolonged centrally generated activation may cause physiological changes associated with increased risk of disease. We have shown that the cortisol response may be a distinguishing feature of activation associated with distressing events. Recent advances in the central neurobiology of cortisol regulation indicate widespread effects of stress levels of cortisol on the central nervous system. These effects are adaptive if they are confined to short-term activation and occasional episodes. The effects of severe and prolonged pituitary-adrenocortical activation are increasingly understood to have deleterious consequences.

In the following chapter, we will consider how challenges encountered in daily life can produce psychological stress responses, and we will examine models of the resulting central nervous system functions leading to autonomic and pituitary adrenocortical activation.

Summary

We have evolved a complex set of physiological controls to maintain homeostasis in the face of physical threats. These controls compensate for physical changes in the external or internal environment. But we can also often experience perceived threats and emotional upsets associated with psychological distress. Psychological stressors affect the state of the body by altering the same mechanisms that we evolved to compensate for physical threats. Exercise is an example of physical stress, and psychomotor tasks and mental arithmetic are examples of psychological stressors commonly used in laboratory research.

The emotional characteristics of these stressors are crucial for determining the pattern of autonomic and endocrine activation. Emotionally positive, activating challenges call forth increased cardiovascular and catecholamine responses without activating cortisol. Emotionally negative, distressed states selectively produce rises in cortisol to accompany the cardiovascular and catecholamine activation. Therefore, cortisol may be specifically sensitive to negative emotional states such as fear. Psychological stress responses are internally generated and affect the body in a top-down fashion. Such responses, often associated with negative emotions, may occur frequently in social settings without being acted out behaviorally. These repeated responses may have negative health consequences.

Further Reading

Charvat, J., Dell, P., & Folkow, B. (1964). Mental factors and cardiovascular diseases. *Cardiologia, 44,* 124–141.

A classic account of the theory that stress can lead to illness.

Folkow, B. (1993). Physiological organization of neurohormonal responses to psychosocial stimuli: Implications for health and disease. *Annals of Behavioral Medicine, 15,* 236–244.

A recent account of integrated stress mechanisms in relation to behavior.

Bear, M. F., Connors, B. W., & Paradiso, M. A. (2001). *Neuroscience: Exploring the brain* (2nd ed.). Baltimore: Lippincott, Williams, & Wilkins.

A useful review of brain systems with information on their impact on the hypothalamic-pituitary-adrenal axis.

Guyton, A. C. (1992). *Human physiology and mechanisms of disease* (3rd ed.). Philadelphia: W. B. Saunders.

An excellent, comprehensive review of human physiology.

Rushmer, R. M. (1989). Structure and function of the cardiovascular system. In N. Schneiderman, P. Kaufmann, & S. Weiss (Eds.), *Handbook of research methods in cardiovascular behavioral medicine* (pp. 5–22). New York: Plenum.

A brief overview of the structure and function of the cardiovascular system.

Weiner, H. (1992). *Perturbing the organism: The biology of stressful experience.* Chicago: University of Chicago Press.

Stanford, S. C., & Salmon, P. (Eds.). (1993). *Stress: From synapse to syndrome.* New York: Academic Press.

Two recent books providing a broad coverage of the field of stress.

6

Central Nervous System Integrations of the Psychological Stress Response

In this chapter, we consider how a person's worldview can influence his or her emotions and thereby cause psychological stress responses. We begin with a functional view of how persons evaluate events and consider how these evaluations may result in negative emotions leading to psychological stress reactions. Negative emotions do not occur in isolation but are part and parcel with particular patterns of brain activity. The discussion will focus on what we know about the neurophysiology of negative affect leading to states of psychological stress. Chapter 4 discussed brain systems underlying the peripheral stress response, with an emphasis on homeostatic regulation based on activities of the hypothalamus, brainstem, and autonomic nervous system. Chapter 5 introduced the idea that stress responses may arise from psychological threats. We now begin to formulate a more complete picture of how psychological events can cause stress reactions. We consider how higher brain systems interact with the regulatory functions of the hypothalamus and brainstem to form psychological stress responses. In so doing, we characterize the process of psychological stress by using functional and neurophysiological models in parallel to understand how psychological responses are tied to events in the brain. This discussion provides further background for our basic question about the ways that ideas can affect the body.

Appraisals, Psychological Stress, and Negative Emotions

Richard Lazarus and Susan Folkman (Folkman, 1984; Lazarus & Folkman, 1984) described how our interactions with the environment may generate emotions that lead to bodily stress responses. They noted that we constantly evaluate the stream of events we encounter. In this appraisal process, we classify events as familiar or unfamiliar and threatening or nonthreatening. Similarly, we generate a stream of behavioral strategies to deal with these unfolding events. Along with these appraisals and behavioral adjustments, we experience emotions that signal us about the success of our behavioral strategies and motivate additional behaviors.

Primary and Secondary Appraisals

Lazarus and Folkman's model of psychological stress takes a cognitive view of how we engage the world. They postulate that we first evaluate events for their threat value. This primary appraisal is intended to ensure that we do not blindly encounter danger but instead recognize it and begin to evolve a plan to deal with it. Next, in a secondary appraisal, we evaluate our options for coping with any presumed threats. This two-level appraisal process determines not only our cognitive and behavioral responses but also our emotional, neurophysiological, autonomic, and endocrine responses to external events. In short, our appraisals determine the nature and magnitude of our psychological reactions and their accompanying physiological adjustments.

Figure 6.1 describes the stages of formulating a psychological stress response. According to Lazarus and Folkman, the main elements entering into our primary appraisal of an event are our beliefs about how the world should work and our commitments to given courses of action. Some events are judged as either benign or irrelevant, and others are perceived as threats or challenges. Events that are classed as benign can be safely ignored and require no special adaptive response. Events are appraised as threatening if they violate our beliefs about the world or block our ability to carry out our commitments in life. When we consider an event a threat, we simultaneously have an emotional reaction that signals alarm and motivates further behavioral and psychological responses along with physiological activation. We then evaluate the variety and availability of coping responses and their effectiveness at reducing or removing the threat.

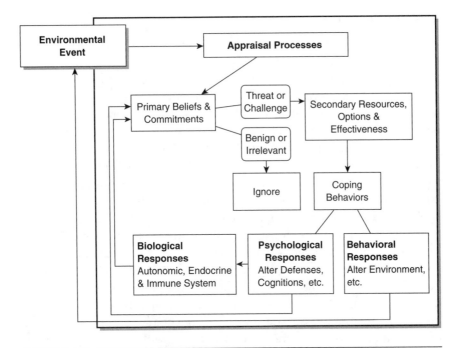

Figure 6.1   Appraisal model of psychological stress. The process of psychological stress includes both primary appraisals of the threat value of an event and secondary appraisals of the effectiveness of available coping options. These two processes have an impact on physiological responses to the situation.

Lazarus's model uses beliefs and commitments as the criteria for deciding what events are threatening. This provides a useful means of accounting for cognitive differences between individuals in emotional responses and stress reactions to a given event. For example, if I fall and break my arm, I may find this event to be inconvenient, painful, and a disruption to my daily life. It is not something I would volunteer for, but I doubt that the misfortune would amount to a personal disaster. On the other hand, imagine this same broken arm happening to an athlete preparing to take part in the Olympic games. In this instance, the broken arm poses a serious threat to the athlete's commitment to a major goal in life. The otherwise manageable inconvenience of wearing a cast for several weeks turns into a devastating event: The athlete has to stop training and may have a severe psychological response, such as depression. Clearly, the same event has different meanings for me and the athlete because of differences in our personal commitments.

Coping Responses

Secondary appraisal focuses appropriately on the kinds of responses that might be employed to manage the event in question, and again, people are likely to differ. Events that are potential or known threats require some adaptive behavioral intervention to ensure that harm is avoided or its negative effects are limited. The interventions we employ are referred to as coping strategies and coping behaviors. These can include both overt and covert activities. If we find ourselves feeling chilly on a winter evening, obvious coping behaviors are to put on a sweater or to turn up the thermostat. But other situations in life are not so obviously correctable, and indeed no simple behavioral strategy may present itself. For example, parents confronted by the news that a young child has a serious, potentially life-threatening illness are likely to receive this as a devastating negative event—one that could have a serious impact on the child and threaten the integrity of the family. This news clearly violates both the beliefs and the commitments that the parents share. However, the most appropriate responses to the situation are difficult to determine because of the complex questions raised: Is the illness curable? What is the effect of the treatment on the child? How long will we have to confront this situation? Will there be financial burdens that may affect other children in the family? How will we manage the added time and energy demands possibly imposed by the situation? There are many potential responses, and all have their costs, strengths, and weaknesses.

In such a complex event as a major illness, the parents may use a multilevel strategy to limit the negative impact on themselves and the rest of the family. Such responses may include learning about the disease to ensure that everything possible is being done for their child and altering their goals and expectations about the course of the child's development and the life of the family. These responses illustrate a combination of adaptive adjustments. Other parents may find themselves overwhelmed by the news and incapable of any directly adaptive response. Instead they may deny that anything is wrong, insisting that the diagnosis is a mistake and even avoiding further treatment for the child. Responses to such a major life stressor may thus involve cognitive approaches to the situation, behavioral adjustments, realignment of goals and commitments, or purely psychological approaches such as denial.

Lazarus and Folkman (1984) have classified coping responses as *problem focused* and *emotion focused*. Problem-focused strategies attack the problem itself, with behaviors designed to gain information, alter the event, and alter beliefs and commitments. Problem-focused strategies increase the person's awareness, level of knowledge, and range of behavioral and cognitive coping options. They can reduce the threat value of the event. Emotion-focused strategies call for psychological changes designed primarily to limit the degree of emotional disruption caused by an event, with minimal effort to alter the event itself.

Outcomes of Coping Efforts and Physiological Responses

As might be expected, each coping strategy has its costs and benefits. Problem-focused strategies may be costly in terms of the energy and time necessary to put them into effect, but they can lessen the stressor value of the event. Emotion-focused strategies are initially less energy consuming but in the long term may be more costly due to a continued drain on coping resources. However, some work suggests that for patients faced with severe cancers, emotion-focused coping, denial in particular, may be stress reducing, whereas problem-focused strategies may be more anxiety provoking (Kreitler, 1999; Watson, Greer, Blake, & Shrapnell, 1984). Whichever style of coping is employed, we strive to reduce the central nervous system activation associated with emotions and to reduce the physiological activation that ensues.

Once a coping strategy has been used, we again evaluate the event in light of our perhaps new beliefs and commitments, and we reassess its threat value. Therefore, the appraisal process is recurrent, and our responses are continuously modified as we deal with the emerging challenges of life. An ultimate goal of the process is to reduce the threat value of events in the environment, reduce the negative emotions in response to them, and therefore reduce the inner responses associated with stress reactions. This process may be seen as a form of cognitive regulation over emotions and states of distress.

In Chapter 5, we noted that fight-or-flight responses are primitive behaviors designed to aid our survival in a physically hostile environment. However, when we encounter events that threaten our beliefs and commitments, we may well find that we experience negative emotions and generate fight-or-flight responses even when our physical well-being is not at stake. Emotional reactions and physiological responses can result from our perceptions of threat from the environment and perceptions of the success of our coping efforts.

Stress responses based on perceptions of threat are considered to be psychological stress responses because the threat value depends largely on our interpretation of the event and its meaning for our own lives. We might say the following things about psychological stressors:

1. They achieve their threat value not from their physical ability to do harm but from their appraised threat value.

2. They are not equally stressful to all persons.

3. Persons will vary in their ability to cope with perceived stressors.

4. The physiological systems we use to respond to psychological stressors are the same ones that react to physical threats to homeostasis.

Some of the psychological stressors described in Chapter 5, such as performing mental arithmetic in a laboratory study, are pure examples of psychologically threatening events. However, for conscious persons, physically threatening events nearly always present a psychological threat as well. Being caught without shelter in a snowstorm will surely challenge the person's homeostatic mechanisms of temperature regulation, but the person is also likely to suffer considerable anxiety and emotional distress due to awareness of the danger to his or her well-being. So we might say that persons conscious of their situation are likely to have significant psychological concomitants to any genuine physical threat.

Lazarus and Folkman (1984) posed their model in cognitive terms, as if each event we encounter during the day were carefully considered and each response selected consciously from a range of options. However, most of our emotional reactions and stress responses do not have this cognitive character. Despite this, the model works equally well if we exchange the language of cognition for the language of Pavlovian conditioning. We could assume that primary appraisals include implicit appraisals enacted via classically conditioned responses developed through prior experience. Similarly, we could think of secondary appraisals as being shaped by the enactment of behaviorally conditioned coping strategies from our experience. Appraisals may therefore be relatively automatic, conditioned responses or highly cognitive, planned ones. Later in this chapter, we will discuss the role of limbic system structures, especially the amygdala, in forming classically conditioned responses and shaping our cognitive processes.

We have emphasized the generation of emotions as a result of appraisals. It is likely that the particular emotion that results from a situation will depend heavily on the specifics of the appraisal process. Lazarus (1991) has described this relationship at some length.

The Lazarus and Folkman (1984) model does not specify how psychological processes of appraisal and coping might link up with physiological outcomes by way of central nervous system processes and peripheral outflow. Nevertheless, it is possible to specify plausible neurophysiological mechanisms for three major stages in this top-down model of psychological stress: primary appraisals, their accompanying emotions and physiological responses, and modulation of these by coping responses.

Central Integration of the Response to Psychological Stress

We now turn to a model illustrating how encounters with threatening events may be incorporated into neurophysiological changes and autonomic and endocrine outflow. In Chapter 4, we reviewed the mechanisms responsible for maintaining homeostasis, with the hypothalamus at the top of this core regulatory system. We recognize that the hypothalamus and brainstem can maintain bodily functions within normal limits and that they also control reflexive and stereotyped behavioral responses. Figure 4.4 showed the integrated "sham rage" response that was organized by the hypothalamus and brainstem. What these parts of the brain cannot do for cats, or people, is perceive and classify something at a distance from the body, consider a behavioral plan to obtain or avoid that thing, and put the plan into execution, using continuous feedback from the environment to adjust behaviors as they are brought into play. These activities require the remainder of the brain, the parts above the hypothalamus that can sense external events and shape responses to them. Because these parts of the brain are necessary for survival in a free-living animal, they must form the highest controls over homeostasis. The cerebral hemispheres are the parts of the brain that we use to form emotional responses to external objects; they develop the motivations that underlie approach and avoidance behaviors. They are also responsible for stress reactions to external stimuli or, in humans, to thoughts and ideas. In other words, they carry out the top-down processes that lead to our psychological stress reactions. We will review these brain areas and their functions in considering how psychological stress responses are formed.

Figure 6.2 is a simplified flow diagram that we will use to guide our discussion of the chain of psychophysiological events that we believe leads from an event in the environment to the generation of a reaction in the body. We can think of five major steps in this chain of events:

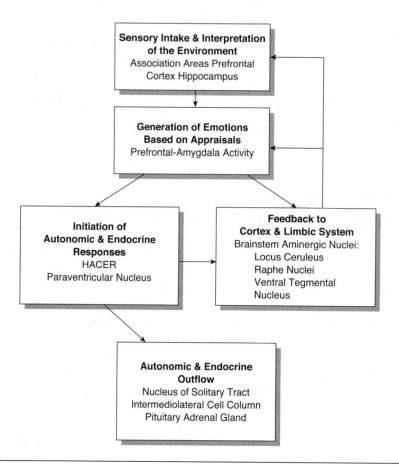

Figure 6.2   Major steps in the generation of physiological responses based on perceptions and interpretations of events.

1. Sensory intake and interpretation of the environment

2. Generation of emotions based on the appraisal processes

3. Initiation of autonomic and endocrine responses

4. Feedback to the cortex and limbic system

5. Autonomic and endocrine outflow

The first four of these steps involve considering how external events affect the regulation of the body. They lead to a consideration of how higher nervous system processes act on the regulatory apparatus involving the hypothalamus and brainstem. As a companion to this simplified diagram, we will review these steps in detail, referring to several related figures that describe areas of the brain and its subsystems.

As we talk about areas of the brain associated with appraisals and the emotions that can lead to stress responses, we will mention brain areas that are shown in Figures 6.3 and 6.4. Figure 6.3 has four views of a human brain with parts of the limbic system and frontal cortex outlined. In view (a), we see the orbital prefrontal cortex, which is the lower surface of the prefrontal cortex, located just above the eyes. Two of its subregions are shown, the medial part and the lateral part. The medial part is the lower portion of the ventromedial prefrontal cortex, also shown in (d). The lateral part is the lateral orbital cortex. View (b) shows the dorso-lateral prefrontal cortex. View (c) shows a slice of the brain indicating where the amygdala is found in the inner convolution of the temporal lobe. Finally, in (d) we can see a view of the middle surface of the brain with the curving anterior cingulate gyrus, which is just above the medial surface of the ventromedial prefrontal cortex.

Figure 6.4a shows the limbic lobe. The term refers to the regions of the cortex that include the parahippocampal gyrus and the cingulate gyrus. The parahippocampal gyrus overlies the hippocampus and amygdala. The cingulate gyrus communicates at each part of its length to adjacent areas of sensory and motor cortex. Finally, information about ongoing sensory processes, motor behaviors, and motivational states is communicated to the anterior part of the cingulate gyrus. The anterior cingulate is closely tied to the functions of the areas of the prefrontal cortex outlined in Figure 6.3. The primary limbic system structures and their inter-connections are shown in Figure 6.4b. The principal connections are from the amygdala to the basal ganglia, including the bed nuclei of the stria terminalis and the nucleus accumbens. The primary pathways from the amygdala are the stria terminalis and ventral amygdalofugal pathway. The second important set of pathways connects the hippocampus to the mammillary bodies by way of the fornix. The limbic system and its con-nections with the cortex help us form motivations to avoid things that are dangerous, approach and obtain things that are needed for survival, and remember motivationally relevant experiences for future reference. In cases of real or perceived danger, the limbic system, especially outputs from the amygdala, is responsible for integrating a state of fight-or-flight. This pattern is the key component of an acute stress reaction. To appre-ciate the development of an acute psychological stress response, it is useful to first consider how information arriving from the environment is processed and interpreted.

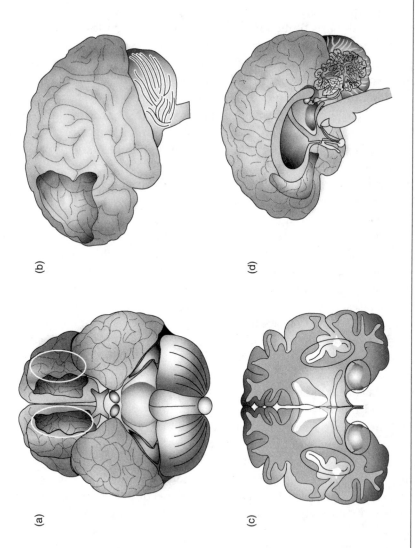

Figure 6.3 Brain areas associated with emotions and evaluations of current events. (a) The orbital prefrontal cortex showing the medial and lateral areas. (b) The dorsolateral prefrontal cortex. (c) The amygdala and insula. (d) The anterior cingulate gyrus just above the ventromedial prefrontal cortex.

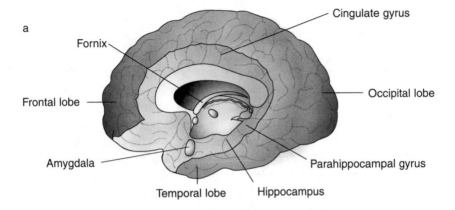

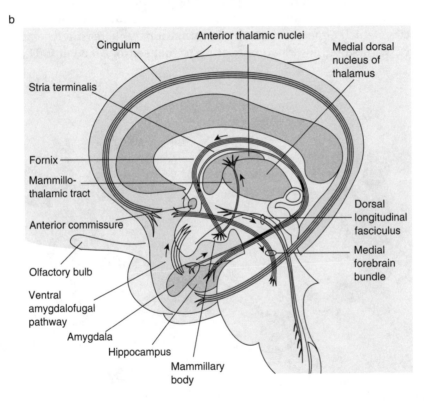

Figure 6.4   The limbic lobe and limbic system with related structures. (a) The areas of cortex collectively known as the limbic lobe. These include the parahippocampal gyrus in the medial temporal lobe, the cingulate gyrus, and ventromedial prefrontal cortex. (b) The limbic system. The amygdala is shown with its major outputs, the stria terminalis and the ventral amygdalofugal pathway terminating at the bed nuclei of the stria terminalis and the nucleus accumbens.

Sensory Intake and
Interpretation of the Environment

Sensory information is relayed to and through the thalamus, which acts as the central way station for most incoming information. The thalamus directs information to the primary cortical projection areas, dedicated to the various sensory modalities. Figure 6.5 illustrates the surface of a brain and indicates the primary visual and auditory projection areas and the pathways by which sensory information travels from these areas. The primary projection area for vision is located at the back of the cortex, and the projection area for auditory sensation is on the upper surface of the temporal lobe. This incoming information passes next through a series of unimodal sensory association areas of the cortex, during which time raw sensory information is increasingly elaborated with stored information relating to that sensory modality. These

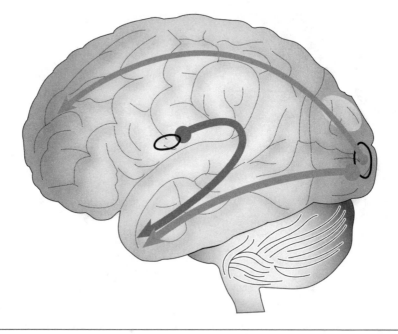

Figure 6.5 Flow of sensory information. Left view of a human brain, showing the flow of visual information, from the occipital cortex, and auditory information, from the superior temporal gyrus, to form polymodal sensory inputs to the inferior temporal cortex. Visual inputs to the frontal lobes are indicated from the occipital cortex.

elaborations are responsible for giving percepts the familiar objectlike qualities that familiar things have.

If someone throws us a red ball, we see a red ball and not just a patch of red moving in our direction. In addition to these unimodal associational processes, we have multisensory experiences. The red ball may fly so close and fast that it makes a swishing sound as it passes. This integrated visual and auditory experience depends on the contribution of polymodal association cortex, parts of the associational areas that combine inputs from more than one unimodal association area. This is illustrated in Figure 6.5, showing the convergence of visual and auditory sensory inputs at the inferior temporal gyrus, an area we will discuss in more detail in connection with the amygdala. For the moment, it is sufficient to think of this as a multisensory superhighway of highly processed associations that is the main source of inputs to specific areas of our limbic systems. A final feature of this diagram is a visual pathway indicated as passing along a different route directed at the ventromedial prefrontal cortex. The prefrontal cortex can be seen as divided into a higher lateral portion, including the ventromedial prefrontal cortex, directed at processing information in a highly cognitive mode, and an inferior portion, including the orbital cortex, which has a greater visceral and motivational representation (see Figure 6.3a and b).

As these higher stages of processing suggest, things initially perceived gain motivational properties as the sensory information gives way to its classification, appraisal, and meaning. To appraise something calls for estimating its nature, quality, or importance. These activities appear to correspond to the primary stages of appraisal outlined by Lazarus, and this process is different from simply perceiving. It is the beginning of taking action, or not, and it calls for neurophysiological processes and structures that differ from purely sensory and associational ones. Here the stream of conscious experience takes on two qualities, one that is purely cognitive and one that is affectively colored. These two qualities of consciousness may well have distinct neural substrates.

On the cognitive side of this equation, the end point is the prefrontal cortex, especially the dorsolateral portion. These prefrontal regions are essential to our ability to attach meaning or significance to the information we receive. On the affective side of the equation are the structures of the temporal lobe, the limbic system, the basal forebrain, or what we will call frontal-limbic connections. We will deal with each of these in turn. The key point here is that the evaluation of events for meaning and significance and then an affective flavor captures the essence of the appraisal process. The appraisal process determines how we form emotions and stress reactions.

Cognition and Emotion: Generating Emotions Based on Appraisal Processes

The appraisal process therefore leads us to consider both the cognitive and the affective side of things in developing a model of events leading up to psychological stress reactions. Before we explore the more affective side, it is worthwhile to consider the cognitive functions of the prefrontal cortex. Figure 6.5 indicates pathways that lead to the frontal lobes, areas of the brain that participate in assessing the meaning and significance of inputs. In relation to appraisal processes, the dorsolateral prefrontal cortex is especially important for our ability to consciously work through complex problems. There is much evidence that this is the area most specialized for working memory (Goldman-Rakic, 1996; Courtney, Petit, Maisog, Ungerleider, & Haxby, 1998). Carrying out arithmetic problems "in our head" and mentally rotating a recalled image of a baseball glove are two examples of working memory tasks. Working memory is a set of processes that allow us direct our attention, allow events to be evaluated in consciousness, and consider alternative courses of action—just the sorts of skills necessary to carry out primary and secondary appraisals.

Frontal lobe functioning, then, is crucial for assessing the meaning of ongoing events. However, purely cognitive processes are not particularly useful in making real decisions. To make effective decisions leading to action in our daily lives, we also need to know how we feel about things. For this reason, the frontal lobes also have abundant visceral inputs that tell our decision-making apparatus how the body is responding as events are experienced and courses of action are considered.

Impressive demonstration of this affective role of the frontal lobes comes from patients who have sustained damage to specific areas of the frontal cortex. The most famous such patient is Phineas Gage (Figure 6.6). As recounted by his physician, John Harlow (1868), Gage was foreman of a blasting crew cutting a new railroad through the mountains of Vermont. His job called for setting black powder charges in holes drilled into the rock by his crewmen. On September 13, 1848, he was briefly distracted while setting a charge, and his iron tamping rod slipped from his hands into the hole his assistant had just filled with a powder charge. The resulting detonation propelled the tamping rod upward and entirely through Gage's skull. The extraordinary aspect of this case is that Gage lost consciousness only for a matter of minutes. He remained lucid at all times. He could describe the accident in detail, and an hour afterward he walked upstairs to his room at a nearby boardinghouse. Testing by Harlow and

RECOVERY

FROM THE

PASSAGE OF AN IRON
BAR THROUGH THE HEAD.

By JOHN M. HARLOW, M.D.,

OF WOBURN.

(With a Plate)

Read June 3, 1868

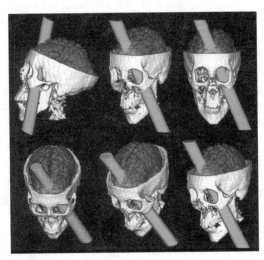

Journal of the Massachusetts Medical Society. 1868;2:327-347

Figure 6.6   The front page of Dr. John Haslow's classic paper on Phineas Gage. Phineas Gage's reconstructed skull and brain. (Skull images reprinted with permission from *Science no. 264, no. 5162 20 May 1994*. Digital image: H Damasio. Copyright © 1994 AAAS.)

others indicated that he was cognitively intact and fully aware of his surroundings. He retained his rational faculties, but, as his friends observed, "Gage was no longer Gage." He had become socially boorish, had lost his social inhibitions, and had lost his previous goal-oriented approach to life. Although he supported himself until his death on May 21, 1861, he became a shiftless drifter, going from one menial job to another. Dr. Harlow, who followed Gage through the remaining 12 years of his life, subsequently donated Gage's skull and the tamping rod to the museum at Harvard College. Through John Harlow's extraordinary writing and an innovative reconstruction of Gage's injury by Hannah Damasio and her colleagues (Damasio, Grabowski, Frank, Galaburda, & Damasio, 1994), who used magnetic resonance imaging techniques for the purpose, we now know that the injury "involved both left and right prefrontal cortices in a pattern that, as confirmed by Gage's modern counterparts, causes a defect in rational decision making and the processing of emotion" (p. 1102). Such patients find it difficult to invest events with meaning and to make informed choices about future actions based on feelings about their consequences.

Insight into Phineas Gage's deficit comes from studies of modern patients with similar lesions. This work is summarized engagingly by Antonio Damasio (1994), who reported that patients with frontal lesions, particularly bilateral damage to the ventromedial prefrontal cortex and related areas, are often fully conscious and able to perform normally on tests of intelligence. But these people are dramatically impaired in making wise decisions. Damasio provides the striking example of a patient with ventromedial prefrontal damage who was given a simple choice of two dates for a follow-up appointment about a month later. Most persons would think for a moment and state a preference for one option. In this case, the patient began a lengthy discussion of each option, rationally stating the pros and cons of each, but in spite of this evaluation, he was unable to decide which date would be better until his physician, in desperation, suggested a date. The patient immediately agreed to that date and happily left the office as if his former monologue was irrelevant! In Damasio's words, "We might conclude that the result of these patients' lesions is the discarding of what their brains have acquired through education and socialization. One of the most distinctive human traits is the ability to learn to be guided by future prospects rather than by immediate outcomes" (p. 218). Such patients are not necessarily devoid of emotional experience. Often they may exhibit emotional reactions that are inappropriate for the time or situation, as did Phineas Gage. What these patients lack is the ability to have normal emotional responses in relation to present thoughts and events.

Prefrontal-Limbic Interactions
and Thoughts and Feelings

How do the functions of the frontal lobes help us understand the processes leading to psychological stress reactions? Antonio Damasio has argued for the importance of the frontal lobes and their connections to limbic structures. It is through these connections that we invest information with meaning and emotional valence. The parts of the prefrontal cortex that are crucial for forming the visceral coloration of thoughts and ideas are the ventromedial prefrontal cortex and the closely associated anterior cingulate gyrus (Figure 6.3d). These areas and their limbic connections, the prefrontal-limbic connections, help us feel about things, not just coldly compare sterile bits of information. This reasoning leads us to place the connections from the limbic system, especially those projecting from the amygdala toward the basal ganglia and the prefrontal cortex, at the beginning of the chain of events resulting in normal emotional responses and perhaps leading to physiological stress responses.

Physiological Correlates of Primary
and Secondary Appraisal Processes

There is a strong parallel between primary appraisals and frontal lobes' processes that allow us to give meaning to events. During secondary appraisals, we must be able to invest alternative coping strategies with both meaning and emotional content in order to choose the best alternative. The addition of emotional content depends on connecting the activity of the prefrontal cortex with other structures specialized for the formation of emotional responses. As illustrated in Figure 6.5, the sensory stream has cognitive and affective components that ultimately are processed in the frontal cortex. The cognitive route depends on relatively direct pathways from sensory areas to the prefrontal cortex. The visceral route involves the inferior temporal lobe, which we may think of as the main point of entry from the amygdala, other parts of the limbic system, and internal bodily sensations. These inputs via the inferior temporal lobe may shape both steps in the appraisal process.

The limbic system is therefore intimately connected to the incoming flow of sensory information, it shapes thoughts and motivations, and it can take control of autonomic centers in the hypothalamus and brainstem when response to external events is required. A consideration of these mechanisms will occupy the rest of this chapter.

The neural structures involved in processing sensory inputs, appraising them, forming emotions, and generating bodily outputs are summarized in Figure 6.7. The right part of the diagram indicates sensory information being processed through successively higher levels of association cortex and the convergence of information at the inferior temporal gyrus, located along the lower surface of the temporal lobe. Here information is passed to the parahippocampal gyrus, located along the medial surface of the temporal lobe. At this point, the highly processed inputs become available to both the hippocampus and the amygdala. These structures have parallel and complementary functions. The hippocampus is associated with the formation of declarative memories, which are memories for facts and events. Damage to, or surgical removal of, the hippocampus will impair or eliminate the person's ability to form new memories of daily experiences. Brenda Milner's reports on the famous patient H.M., who had bilateral surgical removal of his hippocampal regions, dramatically illustrate the devastating impact of such a deficit (Milner & Penfield, 1955; Scoville & Milner, 2000). Even after years of living in a new neighborhood, H.M. was unable to develop a cognitive map of his surroundings and had to be accompanied on walks.

The amygdala performs a parallel memory function. It is essential to the formation of Pavlovian conditioned associations, and in relation to these associations it is essential in forming appropriate motivational states with regard to the external world and our feelings about that world. Recall that in Pavlovian conditioning two types of sensory events come to be associated with each other. According to the usual example, Pavlov's dog was given numerous pairings of a bell sounding and placement of food directly into its mouth via a feeding tube. This involved, therefore, the pairing of a sound, an exteroceptive sensation, with an input from outside the body that became a signal for the next event, which was an interoceptive sensation, coming from the taste and feel of food inside the mouth. Finally, the dog learned to salivate in anticipation of the arrival of food when the bell sounded. We now know that the formation of such associations is impossible if the amygdala is destroyed (Davis & Whalen, 2001). Together, these medial temporal lobe structures appear to be essential to building up a normal repertoire of experiences of external events and their motivational meanings, with the hippocampus allowing us to form the mental representations of events and the amygdala giving these representations their visceral associations.

Research using animal models has indicated the importance of the amygdala in generating appropriate responses to threatening situations. Young primates that have never before seen a snake will back away in

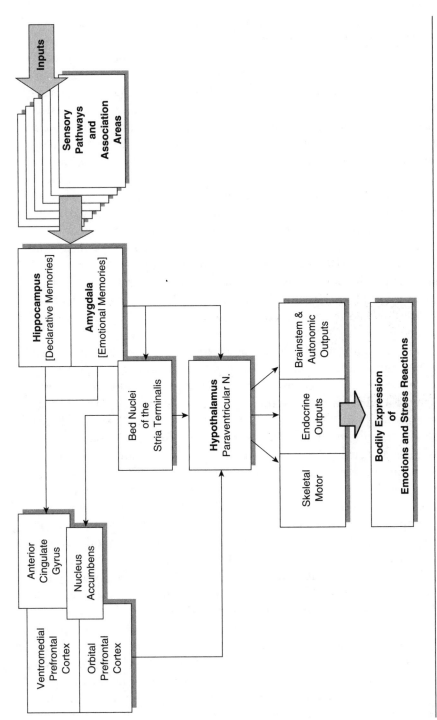

Figure 6.7 Neurophysiologically based model of the primary brain processes determining autonomic and endocrine responses to psychological stress.

extreme fear when a rubber snake is presented at the front of their home cage. This suggests that innate programs are in place to help the animal avoid danger. In contrast, surgically amygdalectomized young animals do not hesitate to approach and explore unfamiliar objects. Young primates who have been amygdalectomized prior to exposure to the rubber snake will readily approach it, pick it up, and handle it. Similarly, amygdalectomized rats will approach and explore a sedated cat, completely lacking their innate avoidance of this predator. Such animals are slow to learn to avoid places where aversive stimulation has occurred or to learn to escape when given cues signaling impending shock. Another, more interpretive way to look at these results is that amygdalectomized animals are deprived of their ability to look forward to potential negative consequences of their behaviors in light of current sensory information. The amygdala helps us form Pavlovian conditioned associations, which form the motivational basis for emotional reactions to the environment and shape our psychological stress responses. This system's ability to shape emotional memories gives us the ability to modify responses to motivationally significant events based on experience. A detailed discussion is provided by Davis (2000).

In its role in forming Pavlovian associations, the amygdala is a point of convergence of information about conditional stimuli, which usually include exteroceptive sensory information, and unconditional stimuli, which most often arise as visceral or tactile sensations. Sensory information arriving from outside the body, notably as visual and auditory inputs, is transmitted to the inferior temporal cortex, while interoceptive sensations are carried to the insular cortex (buried behind the temporal lobe and outlined in Figure 6.3c), the amygdala, and the anterior cingulate gyrus. The hippocampus and the amygdala therefore come to form a critical pair of structures in our neurophysiological model of stress reactions. The hippocampus is essential for recognizing familiar events, and the amygdala is equally essential for forming memories of the emotional connotations of these events as Pavlovian conditioned associations. Does the bell signal the arrival of food or the onset of an electric shock? Clearly, the motivational qualities of the bell will be vastly different in the two cases, and the bodily outputs will correspondingly differ.

The outputs of the hippocampus and amygdala therefore appear to be essential for appropriate interpretations and formation of coping responses. Figure 6.7 indicates a pair of pathways from the hippocampus and amygdala to the anterior cingulate gyrus. The anterior cingulate gyrus is active in animals that are choosing among behavioral alternatives under motivational conditions. This merging of hippocampal and amygdaloid inputs builds upon the hippocampus's role of registering contextual information and the amygdala's role of providing motivational value to specific cues, both pieces of information being important in making informed behavioral choices or selecting coping strategies. A second set of connections in Figure 6.7 shows outputs from the amygdala to the bed nuclei of the stria terminalis (which occur two on each side of the brain) and then to the closely associated nucleus accumbens. These sets of structures are located beneath the surface of the rear part of the ventromedial prefrontal cortex, near where it is joined by the anterior cingulate gyrus (Figures 6.3d and 6.4b). Therefore, this appears to be an area where sensory inputs acquire motivational significance. We might also think of it as an area where the dialogue between experience and emotion is carried out. The diagram shows the areas representing the prefrontal cortex, nucleus accumbens, and anterior cingulate gyrus as overlapping—a visual shorthand indicating that the interconnections are extensive. Recalling the specific consequences for patients with damage to the area where the anterior cingulate gyrus meets the ventromedial prefrontal cortex, we understand more clearly that forming appropriate behavioral strategies is dependent on the provision of higher centers such as the ventromedial prefrontal cortex with this essential information about context, motivational value, and response alternatives.

Recent gains in understanding the neurophysiology of the frontal lobes show the extent of the connections from these areas to the limbic system by way of the basal ganglia. Figure 6.8 indicates two such pathways. Both loops involve inputs from the thalamus to the frontal cortex. The loops are closed by outputs from the frontal areas, through different parts of the basal ganglia, back to the thalamus. The left loop is modulated by inputs from the hippocampus that influence inputs from the thalamus to the dorsolateral prefrontal cortex. This loop would appear specialized for processing information in working memory in view of current inputs processed by the hippocampus. The right loop involves inputs from the central nucleus of the amygdala that engage pathways from the thalamus to the anterior cingulate gyrus by way of the nucleus accumbens. Disruption of either or both of these pathways, as in the case of Phineas Gage's injury, would have a marked effect on the sources of information available to areas of the frontal lobes involved in making decisions and choosing among alternative strategies. We refer to the higher pathways outlined in Figures 6.7 and 6.8 with the shorthand term *frontal-limbic*, indicating that they bring together processes associated with the emotions and processes we think of as purely cognitive.

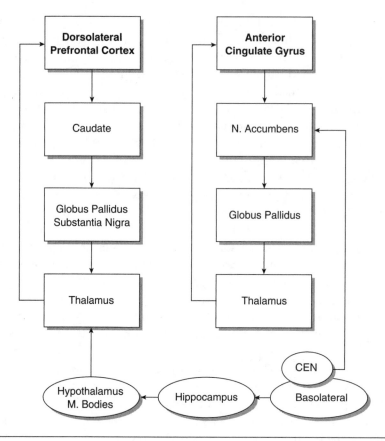

Figure 6.8   Frontal connections to basal ganglia. One loop shows the involvement of the hippocampus in modulating activity involving the dorsolateral prefrontal cortex. The other loop involves the amygdala and outputs to the nucleus accumbens affecting communication to the anterior cingulate gyrus.

These frontal-limbic interactions are likely to be critical for both primary and secondary appraisals as outlined in Lazarus and Folkman's (1984) model of psychological stress. Primary appraisals involve recognizing if something is dangerous. Secondary appraisals involve reviewing the available coping responses, evaluating a plan of action, and examining possible outcomes in view of their costs and benefits. The frontal-limbic connections specified in our model suggest that the psychological processes postulated by Lazarus and Folkman have reasonable neurophysiological candidates.

Sources of Amygdaloid Activity and Internally Generated Emotional Responses

We have spoken of psychological stressors as if they always began as external events. But we all know from personal experience that some of the most consistent sources of psychological distress are our own thoughts and ruminations. Jay Schulkin, Bruce McEwen, and Phil Gold (1994) have described how we may agonize over future events or past actions and how such distressing mental activity may generate the same frontal-limbic responses that would occur if we were confronting a genuine external threat. These recalled or imagined events are certainly able to engage the limbic system and the related bodily outputs. Understanding the frontal-limbic mechanisms underlying the generation of emotions helps us appreciate the very close association between our abilities to evaluate the world, formulate coping strategies, and shape our emotional experience.

Initiation of Behavioral, Autonomic, and Neuroendocrine Responses to Psychological Stressors

The next steps in the model concern how our appraisals and associated emotions lead to changes in our peripheral physiology by way of autonomic and endocrine outputs. Considering the amygdala's position in the path of sensory input and its extensive connections to frontal areas and to the hypothalamus and brainstem, we may say that the amygdala is a focal point where information arriving as sensory inputs is first tagged with affective coloration and where autonomic and endocrine responses begin to be formulated. Figure 6.7 indicates that the hypothalamus is a point of convergence of inputs from the amygdala (directly, but mainly via the bed nuclei of the stria terminalis) and the orbital prefrontal cortex. In addition, some of these pathways pass through the hypothalamus and descend directly to the upper brainstem, notably the pons and medulla. Figure 6.4b shows the location of the major pathway that makes these frontal-brainstem connections, the medial forebrain bundle.

The outputs of the hypothalamus and their engagement with the brainstem account for skeletal motor, autonomic, and endocrine expressions of emotions and stress responses. The skeletal motor patterns are incorporated as complex reflex programs and are responsible, to give one example, for the motor components of the sham rage exhibited by Cannon and Bard's decerebrate cats (Bard, 1928). The endocrine outputs will be discussed in Chapter 7. The autonomic outputs associated with states of fight-or-flight are generated by nuclei of the brainstem with inputs from the hypothalamus.

The brainstem pons and medulla incorporate two functional subsystems. The first is the central feedback subsystem, which includes the pontine reticular formation and its aminergic nuclei. This subsystem serves to regulate the functional state of the entire central nervous system, causing it to switch gears to meet behavioral emergencies and also to become quiescent when appropriate. The second subsystem is the brainstem response subsystem, which includes the descending pathways that arrive at the muscles and viscera of our bodies. They include the nucleus paragigantocellularis, the nucleus of the solitary tract, and the intermediolateral cell column. This subsystem also has feedback loops to and from the viscera, allowing reflex control over autonomic responses.

Feedback to the Cortex and Limbic System: The Central Feedback Subsystem

Once incoming information has been categorized and appraised and an initial response has been formulated, it may be important to reset the state of the central nervous system to act entirely in concert to meet a serious threat or to attain a highly desirable goal. This is accomplished by a network of nuclei in the brainstem that we may think of as the central feedback subsystem because it provides feedback to the central nervous system about its own activities. The central feedback subsystem consists of the reticular formation and three specialized components, the aminergic nuclei. This subsystem determines the global behavioral state of the person. Depending on commands from the amygdala and hypothalamus, it can prepare us to meet an emergency if we need to respond to one, or it can put us to sleep if it is safe to do so. Its functions are not simply activational, however. This system's outputs to frontal-limbic areas determine our threshold for experiencing positive and negative affect in given situations. They also determine our longer-term sense of well-being or dysphoria.

The pontine reticular formation is a diffuse collection of fibers and specialized nuclei. It is phylogenetically very old, and in primitive species it connects sensory systems with systems allowing the formation of behavioral and physiological responses. It plays a similar role in humans, with considerably greater integration and control from higher centers, especially motor and decision-making systems controlled by the cortex.

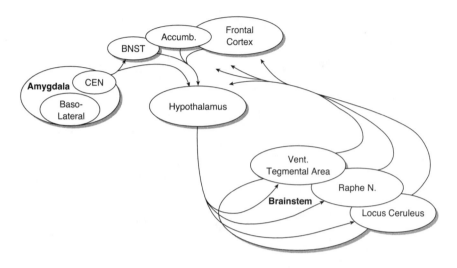

Figure 6.9   The central feedback subsystem. The outputs from the central nucleus of the amygdala (CEN) to the bed nucleus of the stria terminalis (BNST) and nucleus accumbens (Accumb.) and descending pathways to and through the hypothalamus to the brainstem aminergic nuclei. The ascending projections are directed to all parts of the cerebral hemispheres, with especially heavy representation to hypothalamus and frontal-limbic areas.

The aminergic nuclei contain cell bodies that synthesize the monoamine neurotransmitters: norepinephrine, serotonin, and dopamine. Figure 6.9 schematizes the inputs and outputs from these nuclei. In general, their inputs arise from frontal-limbic areas and indirectly from the amygdala by way of the bed nuclei of the stria terminalis. In turn, these nuclei send fibers to all parts of the central nervous system to set our behavioral state. These small groupings of cell bodies are therefore extremely important in determining the state of the entire cortex and in shaping the interplay of emotional experience, brain states, and autonomic and motor outflow. Each set of nuclei has a different neurotransmitter. The locus ceruleus contains norepinephrine fibers, the raphe nuclei have serotonin neurons, and the ventral tegmental area has neurons that produce dopamine.

In addition, each set of nuclei and their accompanying transmitter systems perform different but complementary functions. The locus ceruleus contains 90% of the norepinephrine-synthesizing cell bodies in the central nervous system, and these send fibers to the cortex, limbic structures, and spinal cord, as indicated in Figure 6.10 (Aston-Jones,

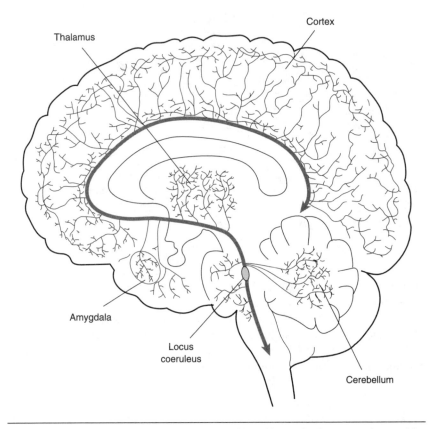

Figure 6.10   Projections of noradrenergic fibers from the locus ceruleus to the rest of the central nervous system. (Adapted with permission from "Volume Transmission in the Brain," by L. F. Agnati, B. Bjelke, and K. Fuxe, 1992, *American Scientist, 80,* 362–373.)

Ennis, Pieribone, Nickell, & Shipley, 1986). The norepinephrine fiber system functions most clearly as the brain's global arousal system. This area is highly active during highly aroused behavioral states, such as states of fight-or-flight, and it is nearly silent during deep stages of sleep. Figure 6.10 will provide an appreciation of how a small nucleus containing only a few thousand cell bodies, such as the locus ceruleus, can affect the activational state of the entire central nervous system.

The raphe nuclei have serotonin-containing fibers that ascend to frontal-limbic areas, including the amygdala, the hypothalamus, and areas of the anterior cingulate gyrus and orbital prefrontal cortex. It is noteworthy that affective balance and mood disorders are strongly associated with the functioning of this system. Several major psychoactive medications, particularly antidepressants, act on the serotonin transmitter system. So we globally associate this system with long-term regulation of affect, and its dysregulation with mood disorders.

The ventral tegmental area is a major source of the brain's dopaminergic fibers that project upward to the cortex. This system seems to modulate the processing of incoming information, and altered dopaminergic function is implicated in the symptoms of schizophrenia. Dopamine is released in the nucleus accumbens during the euphoria associated with drug intake (Comings & Blum, 2000) and in response to playing a thrilling video game (Koepp et al., 1998). The dopaminergic system also affects our moods over the long term. For these reasons, the dopaminergic system is thought to generate the experience of pleasure associated with states of reward. Clearly, it influences how we process incoming information and shapes affective responses, especially positively hedonic aspects of our experience (Blum, Cull, Braverman, & Comings, 1996).

Since the aminergic nuclei receive abundant inputs directly or indirectly from the amygdala, we might expect them to be sensitive to negative mood states. This is the case. For example, reduced norepinephrine in the locus ceruleus has been implicated in animal models of depression. Similarly, reduced function of the raphe nuclei, shown by low serotonin levels, is associated with defective social interactions and increased hostility and violent behavior (Brown, Goodwin, Ballenger, Goyer, & Major, 1986). Persons deficient in dopaminergic receptors are also characteristically more irritable than those with a greater receptor density. We will say more about the locus ceruleus and raphe nuclei in Chapter 8, but we can see that the amygdala, acting directly on these nuclei, can alter the functional state of the central nervous system and organize responses appropriate to such negative moods.

The central feedback subsystems associated with the brainstem aminergic nuclei therefore serve to coordinate the level of arousal and the affective tone and behavioral state of the entire central nervous system in response to the commands of the amygdala and of frontal-limbic processes. We can think of them as bringing the separate elements in the central nervous system into line, whether the situation calls for fight-or-flight, approach, avoidance, or sleep.

Autonomic and Endocrine Outflow: The Brainstem Response Subsystem

In accordance with the role of the hypothalamus and brainstem as way stations to the body, the outputs described above have extensive influence

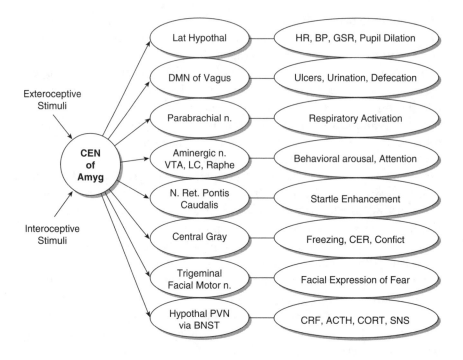

Figure 6.11 The outputs from the central nucleus of the amygdala (CEN) to hypothalamus and brainstem with ultimate effects on peripheral physiology. Key: BNST = bed nucleus of the stria terminalis, HR = heart rate, BP = blood pressure, GSR = galvanic skin response, CER = conditioned emotional responses, CRF = corticotropin releasing factor, ACTH = adrenocorticotropin, CORT = cortisol, SNS = sympathetic nervous system, n. = nucleus, DMN = dorsal motor nucleus of the vagus nerve, PVN = paraventricular nucleus of the hypothalamus, LC = locus ceruleus, VTA = ventral tegmental area.

on a large number of response systems involved in the emotions and stress responses. Figure 6.11 indicates the extensive role played by the amygdala in shaping bodily outputs associated with the emotions and states of stress. Michael Davis (2000) has summarized many anatomical and neurophysiological studies that show a central role for the amygdala in a wide range of bodily expressions of the emotions. The pathways from the central nucleus of the amygdala arrive directly or indirectly at two areas of the hypothalamus, the lateral hypothalamus and the paraventricular nucleus (PVN).

The lateral hypothalamus is a key area for sympathetic outflow to regions of the brainstem. More descriptive of this area is the term *HACER* (the Hypothalamic Area Controlling Emotional Responses, pronounced ah-SEHR), coined by Orville Smith (see Smith, DeVito, & Astley, 1982). The HACER corresponds anatomically to the lateral portion of the hypothalamus in the area surrounding the fornix. This area affects heart rate, blood pressure, and pupillary dilation, all components of the sympathetic part of the acute fight-or-flight response. Studies in rats and primates have shown that autonomic responses to aversive events, including threat of capture or electric shock, are absent when the areas corresponding to the HACER have been destroyed. However, the behavioral correlates of threat, such as muscular tensing and facial grimacing, are present, indicating that the animal is aware of the impending threat and is experiencing the event appropriately. What appears to be missing are important links to physiological outputs to the periphery. In such animals, the usual cardiovascular changes associated with such threats are greatly diminished. The term *HACER* is used rather than more traditional anatomical designations because several hypothalamic nuclei are involved, and the collection does not correspond directly to a single anatomical designation.

As for other hypothalamic targets of the central nucleus of the amygdala, the PVN will be discussed in more detail in Chapter 7. Areas of the brainstem illustrated in Figure 6.11 are the dorsal motor nucleus of the vagus, which regulates parasympathetic outputs to the visceral organs. The other nuclei listed affect skeletal motor components of emotional states and stress responses. The aminergic nuclei are also shown.

Summary

In this chapter, we have considered how our perceptions of the world and of our ability to cope with challenges in our environment can become the basis for emotional states. Through primary and secondary appraisals, we begin to formulate our physiological responses to psychologically stressful events. Chapter 5 described the layers of control we can use to maintain physiological homeostasis. We can use our higher cognitive functions, involving frontal areas of the cerebral cortex, to evaluate external events in conjunction with critical structures of the limbic system. These evaluative processes form the basis for emotions and also for the formulation of behavioral, autonomic, and endocrine responses to threatening events. We may therefore think of these psychological processes as exerting the highest level of control over our homeostatic functions. More generally, we may think of the appraisal process and its effects on stress responses as central to our basic question of how ideas can come to have power over our bodies.

Further Reading

Lazarus, R. S., & Folkman, S. (1984). *Stress, appraisal and coping*. New York: Springer.

Lazarus, R. S. (1991). *Emotion and adaptation*. New York: Oxford University Press.

There is a large literature on coping processes, psychological stress, and health. Lazarus and Folkman (1984) present a valuable, extended consideration of coping processes and psychological stress. Lazarus (1991) presents an extensive update of his views on emotion in relation to appraisals, coping processes, and adaptive behavior.

Courtney, S. M., Petit, L., Maisog, J. M., Ungerleider, L. G., & Haxby, J. V. (1998). An area specialized for spatial working memory in human frontal cortex. *Science, 279,* 1347–1351.

Evidence that specific regions of the dorsolateral prefrontal cortex serve different kinds of working memory tasks. The paper notes that these areas are shifted more posteriorly in humans than in other primates. The authors speculate that the presence in humans of processes such as planning and intentionality may account for the anatomical reorientation of these functions.

Damasio, A. R. (1994). *Descartes' error: Emotion, reason, and the human brain.* New York: G. P. Putnam's Sons.

A rich account of the clinical consequences of frontal lobe damage and the importance of prefrontal areas for evaluative processes.

Smith, O. A., & DeVito, J. L. (1984). Central neural integration for the control of autonomic responses associated with emotion. *Annual Review of Neuroscience, 7,* 43–65.

A well-integrated account of the organization of higher influences on autonomic outflow in relation to the emotions.

7

Stress and the Endocrine System

The previous chapter discussed central nervous system origins of psychological stress responses. This picture is incomplete without a consideration of central regulation of endocrine functions, endocrine outflow, and especially the effects of endocrine feedback during and after responses to acute stressors. We focus here on the two primary stress hormones, cortisol and epinephrine. These act in concert with all the peripheral components of the acute response to stress, play key roles in how the central nervous system is influenced in reaction to stress responses, and ultimately shape our long-term responsivity to stress. In this discussion, we deal with controls over outgoing stress endocrine messengers, endocrine feedback to the central nervous system, long-term regulation of the stress response, and the formation of both declarative and emotional memories. This will set the stage for our discussions in Chapter 9 on determinants of stress reactivity and in Chapter 10 on ways that early experience can set the nervous system's level of stress reactivity across the life of the organism.

Overview of Stress Endocrine Regulation

Figure 6.7 showed three sets of outputs from the hypothalamus and brainstem that shape bodily stress responses. One output is to the endocrine system, involving control over peripheral-gland secretions that participate in stress reactions. By acting in concert, cortisol and epinephrine bind together actions of separate organs and systems to coordinate wide-spread elements of the peripheral stress response. If we consider the central integration of the endocrine response to stress, we recognize that this response has two components, *feed-forward* processes and *feedback* processes. The feed-forward processes, discussed in Chapter 6, determine the magnitude and patterning of autonomic and endocrine activity that affects the periphery. These processes arise from the frontal-limbic inter-actions that impinge on the hypothalamus and brainstem and addition-ally from the coordinating actions of the brainstem aminergic nuclei as these send activational messages back upstream to the brain. The hor-monal feedback processes associated with the stress endocrine system regulate (a) short-term secretion of stress hormones themselves; (b) gene expression in frontal-limbic areas that modulate long-term stress respon-sivity; and (c) shaping of memories for emotionally significant events and consequently altered appraisal processes. Feedback to frontal-limbic areas and the shaping of memories can have long-term influences on which stimuli gain significance for the person in the future and thus determine the extent of bodily response to those stimuli. We will start by describing the core of the stress endocrine system, how it is activated, and how it is regulated by negative feedback.

Activation of Stress Endocrine Secretion and the Central Corticotropin Releasing Factor System

The hypothalamic-pituitary-adrenocortical axis (HPAC) was outlined in Chapter 4. That presentation emphasized the *classical negative feedback model* of glucocorticoid regulation as seen during nonstressful diurnal and metabolic signals (Dallman, 1993). Diurnal signals from the body's clock, the suprachiasmatic nucleus of the hypothalamus, activate the paraven-tricular nucleus of the hypothalamus (PVN) in relation to sleep cycles and glucose regulation, causing variations in the release of corticotropin releasing factor (CRF) to the anterior pituitary, resulting in production of adrenocorticotropin (ACTH) and beta-endorphin, ACTH circulation to the adrenal cortex, and release of cortisol into the systemic circulation (Buijs, van Eden, Goncharuk, & Kalsbeek, 2003). In turn, cortisol secretion is regulated by negative feedback to the pituitary gland via the systemic circulation and to the hypothalamus and hippocampus by way of the cerebrospinal fluid of the ventricles. The net effect is to reduce the secre-tion of both CRF and ACTH. However, during states of stress, regulation differs from this normal pattern, altering both feed-forward and feedback dynamics of HPAC. The feed-forward processes are enhanced, and the feedback is less effective.

Our analysis of how the brain generates bodily responses during psychological stress requires taking a second look at how fight-or-flight states are organized, this time with an emphasis on the roles of CRF and stress hormones. In Chapter 6, we discussed the role of appraisal processes in relation to frontal-limbic activity during the production of affective states and stress responses. We referred to the extensive involvement of the central nucleus of the amygdala in acting on all of the major response systems associated with stress, states of fight-or-flight, and the emotions. We also made special reference to the brain-stem feedback subsystem and how brain activity patterns could be brought into concerted action by the ascending actions of the brainstem aminergic nuclei. We left out one major target of the central feedback subsystem, the *corticotropin releasing factor system.* This is a specialized system of neurons that synthesize CRF and act together to integrate the central nervous system response to stress. Although CRF was initially identified as the hypothalamic neuropeptide responsible for regulation of the HPAC (see Figure 4.5), more recent evidence shows that CRF also acts as a peptide transmitter in a widespread system of neurons that appear to integrate sensory information with states of emotion and the behaviors and to shape autonomic and hormonal responses that accompany these emotions. Portions of the central CRF neuron system are shown in Figure 7.1.

The greatest single accumulation of neurons with CRF-producing cell bodies is found, not surprisingly, in the PVN of the hypothalamus. Some of these cells project to the median eminence of the hypothalamus and others to the brainstem and the spinal cord, where they can modulate autonomic outflow and other functions. A short list of the CRF fiber targets and their functions is given in Table 7.1. In fact, the primary integration of output signals to the cardiovascular and endocrine components of the fight-or-flight response is through these CRF cells of the PVN that project to the median eminence and to the brainstem (Jansen, Nguyen, Karpitskiy, Mettenleiter, & Loewy, 1995).

Other major accumulations of CRF cell bodies are found in the pre-frontal, insular, and cingulate gyrus areas of the cerebral cortex and in the amygdala and hippocampus. As discussed below, the CRF-synthesizing neurons found in these frontal-limbic areas are important for integrating emotions into the central nervous system's formulation of behavioral and physiological stress responses. In Figure 7.1, we give precedence to the

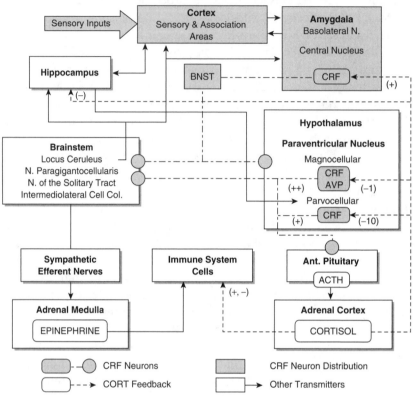

Figure 7.1 The corticotropin releasing factor (CRF) system. The core of the hypothalamic-pituitary-adrenocortical system is shown in the lower right part of the figure. The paraventricular nucleus is shown containing two populations of neurons that synthesize CRF: CRF only and CRF-AVP (arginine vasopressin). CRF-AVP cells exert greater effect on the pituitary than CRF alone (deBold, 1984). The negative feedback of cortisol is 10 times more effective on CRF-only cells than on CRF-AVP cells. The CRF-AVP cells project to the brainstem to activate fight-or-flight–related activities of the autonomic nervous system and stress-related posture and locomotion. A second set of CRF neurons is shown in the central nucleus of the amygdala and the bed nuclei of the stria terminalis (BNST). Projections from the BNST act on the brainstem and lateral hypothalamus and paraventricular nucleus. The cortex, amygdala, and BNST all have significant numbers of CRF cells. Cortisol acts on all cell types in the periphery and the CNS. The figure indicates that epinephrine and cortisol act on immune system cells. One effect of these actions is that cytokines are released. These act indirectly to influence the CNS, notably to increase CRF-AVP secretion by the hypothalamus.

Table 7.1   Brainstem Targets of the Central CRF System Projections From the Hypothalamus and Amygdala

Brainstem CRF Target	Functions of Targets
Locus ceruleus	Source of most noradrenergic cells projecting to the rest of the central nervous system. Activation and coordination of CNS functions. May act to stimulate the extrahypothalamic central CRF system. Antinociception.
Nucleus paragigantocellularis	Programmed outputs associated with emotion-related postures and locomotion.
Periacqueductal gray area	Integrates behaviors with autonomic responses during significant events, especially during fight-or-flight. Enhanced startle during amygdala activation. Antinociception.
Nucleus of the solitary tract	The major autonomic integrating center in the brainstem. Receives inputs from all of the visceral sensory nerves, especially the vagus. This information is distributed to autonomic nuclei and higher centers, including hypothalamus and amygdala. Sends inputs to periacqueductal gray area.
Intermediolateral cell column	Descending outputs to the sympathetic nervous system.

CRF cell bodies of the central nucleus of the amygdala because these cells form primary outputs to the hypothalamus and brainstem and frontal-limbic areas, and these in turn project to the aminergic nuclei of the brainstem. These hypothalamic and brainstem connections have far-reaching consequences for integrating the central nervous system response to negative emotions and stress.

The central CRF system is uniquely and primarily concerned with shaping the feed-forward outputs from the central nervous system to the body during acute states of fight-or-flight. This integrative and highly focused purpose is seen in the CRF system's spatial secretory characteristics, the anatomical distribution of CRF neurons in critical frontal-limbic areas, and the dual endocrine and sympathetic activational properties of CRF neurons in the hypothalamus and brainstem. As Petrusz and Merchenthaler (1992) put it,

> [R]ecent results identify the CRF-41 neuronal system as a widespread and complex system that appears to be dedicated, perhaps uniquely among chemically defined neurons, to a single task: the regulation and coordination of the body's endocrine, autonomic, metabolic, behavioral, and emotional responses to stressful stimuli. (p. 169)

Cortisol's Actions at the Central Nervous System

Cortisol acts on two types of receptors in the central nervous system: *Type I receptors* (also termed mineralocorticoid receptors, or MR) and *Type II receptors* (known as glucocorticoid receptors, or GR). Type I receptors are sensitive to low levels of cortisol and are responsible for cortisol's negative feedback regulation over the diurnal cycle and in response to normal metabolic glucose demands. Type II receptors are about 10 to 20 times less sensitive to cortisol, indicating that they can detect cortisol only when it is present at high levels, making their response sensitivity appropriate to the high cortisol concentrations present during periods of stress. The location and number of each type of receptor in the rat brain are presented in Table 7.2. Several features of this receptor distribution are noteworthy. The hippocampus contains the most receptors and has an almost equal distribution of Type I and II. The amygdala has a much higher number of Type II receptors and a relative absence of Type I. The PVN has both receptor types.

We have discussed cortisol's actions at the central nervous system in terms of negative feedback regulation as it regulates its own secretion and controls stress-related activation. However, the presence of two types of receptors for cortisol, and a wide distribution outside the hypothalamus, suggests that cortisol's actions on the central nervous system are perhaps more complex than just this negative feedback regulation. We earlier described cortisol's functions as both permissive and regulatory (Munck et al., 1984). Cortisol not only permits things to happen when available at low levels but causes other things to happen when present in high quantities. Some appreciation for the effects of cortisol at higher brain centers can be gained by considering the effects of cortisol deficiency and excess.

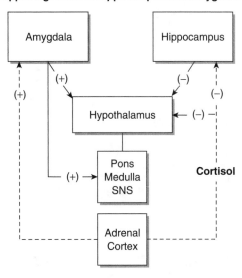

Opposing Roles of Hippocampus and Amygdala

Figure 7.2   The opposing roles of hippocampus and amygdala. The hippocampus exerts primarily tonic restraint on the hypothalamus. In turn, cortisol acts at the hippocampus by negative feedback. The amygdala exerts primarily activational effects on the hypothalamus and brainstem. Cortisol feedback effects are primarily activating at the amygdala.

Adrenalectomized animals and humans with adrenal deficiency have altered sensory thresholds and impairments of learning and memory. In contrast, humans with too much cortisol, due to pituitary tumors or severe depression, have both cognitive and mood disturbances, and these symptoms abate when the tumor is removed or the depression treated with antidepressants (Dorn et al., 1997). Not surprisingly, the places that are most active feedback sites for cortisol are the ones with the most CRF neurons. Areas having high concentrations of CRF-synthesizing neurons include the prefrontal cortex, both its ventrolateral and orbitofrontal regions; the anterior cingulate gyrus; the insular cortex; and the hippocampus and amygdala. Therefore, cortisol feedback regulates its secretion by acting at the hippocampus and PVN. However, through its actions on Type II receptors, stress levels of cortisol appear to be able to modulate functions in all of the higher areas responsible for appraisals of ongoing events and the generation of emotions in response to these.

Table 7.2   Distribution of Adrenal Steroid Receptors in Rat Brain

Region	Type I	Type II	Total	%
Hippocampus	414	305	719	45
Lateral septum	51	194	245	15
Nucl. of solitary tract	76	123	199	13
Central amygdala	9	112	121	8
Locus ceruleus	41	75	116	7
Paraventricular nucl.	28	59	87	6
Supraoptic nucl.	0	60	60	4
Raphe nucl.	0	44	44	3

Note: Regions were punched out from frozen sections of brains of rats perfused at sacrifice with saline. Data represent B max (fmoles/mg protein) from Scatchard analyses. KD to CORT Type 1: 0.5–1 nM; Type 2: 3–5 nM.

Amygdala Responses to Cortisol and Altered Responsivity of the Central Nervous System

Stress levels of cortisol, acting on Type II receptors, can lead to an increased reactivity of the HPAC to stressor presentation. Type II receptors can alter the expression of specific genes in cells that they occupy. This altered gene expression can have long-term and pervasive effects depending on the genes in question and the cell types involved. For our purposes, the most important effect of high levels of cortisol feedback to the central nervous system is on the central nucleus of the amygdala. When cortisol levels are high, repeatedly elevated, or greatly prolonged, the amygdala becomes highly sensitized to any stimulus that is a signal for actual or impending stressor exposure. As a result, high levels of stress actually increase stress reactivity.

An important study in rats illustrates the effect of stress cortisol levels on brain function and behavior. To mimic the effects of stress on the amygdala, investigators implanted corticosterone, the rat version of cortisol, adjacent to the central nuclei of the amygdala in a group of rats, while controls received the surgery but no corticosterone (Shepard, Barron, & Myers, 2000, 2003). One week later, the rats in both groups had normal diurnal patterns of corticosterone secretion, showing that the hypothalamic regulation of secretion was undisturbed. The rats were then exposed to a standard anxiety-provoking stimulus, consisting of an elevated maze with a clear floor and open sides. Circulating corticosterone measurements showed that both groups had equally large acute stress responses, indicating normal initiation of the reaction to this threatening situation. Although this corticosterone response diminished rapidly in the control group, it failed to do so in the corticosterone-exposed rats. Instead, corticosterone output increased steadily until the last blood sample was taken 90 minutes later. In addition, the groups behaved differently on the elevated maze, with implanted rats having much less exploratory activity and showing other behavioral signs of anxiety. Examination of the rats' brains indicated that the implanted rats had greater expression of genes for CRF in the central nuclei of the amygdala, with more neurons expressing CRF and more CRF granules per neuron. In the PVN of the hypothalamus, CRF content of neurons was elevated prior to the stress. In addition, the stressor led to a substantial increase in AVP-gene expression in the PVN of the implanted rats, but no such response occurred in the control rats.

The results suggest some preliminary conclusions. First, the changes in stress sensitivity were specific to the effect of cortisol at the amygdala because the implants were made directly at that site in favor of systemic injections. Second, the increased CRF-gene expression at the amygdala influenced many targets of the central nucleus that determine emotional and behavioral reactions (see Figure 6.10). Third, cortisol at the amygdala resulted in increased stresslike production of AVP at the PVN of the hypothalamus, greatly enhancing ACTH and cortisol production (DeBold et al., 1984, 1987). Fourth, the rats were never subjected to any physically noxious stimuli. They were placed in an open, elevated place, a situation that rats interpret as dangerous, and their reaction appears to be psychologically determined. We can summarize by saying that when the amygdala is exposed to high levels of cortisol, it becomes sensitized to stimuli of a psychologically threatening nature. The consequent increase in CRF gene expression there renders the entire central nervous system highly reactive to fight-or-flight situations. Schulkin et al. (1998) have discussed a range of implications derived from the stress-sensitizing role of high levels of glucocorticoid feedback to the brain.

Amygdala Sensitization and Implications for Health

This amygdala-sensitization model suggests avenues for improved research on human disorders, especially psychosomatic conditions that have long been suspected of having emotional and stress-related contributions. One such disorder is irritable bowel syndrome, which is characterized by frequent gastrointestinal distress, usually following meals, often exacerbated by periods of stress, and unaccompanied by any known organic pathology. Greenwood et al. (2001) tested the amygdala-implant technique in a rat model of bowel pain sensitivity. Their corticosterone-implanted rats became anxiety prone and were more pain sensitive than controls when given a standardized bowel distention test often used in irritable bowel research. Assuming that this test in rats supports an amygdala-based model of anxiety as a contributor to human irritable bowel syndrome, there are interesting clinical connections to stress and irritable bowel in humans. The disorder affects primarily women in the U.S. population, by a 4:1 ratio to men. Half of patients with irritable bowel have psychological distress or psychiatrically diagnosable disorders, many reporting physical or sexual abuse in their past. This research, in relation to the epidemiology of human irritable bowel syndrome, leads to the question of whether a stress sensitivity has been induced in a portion of patients by traumatic life experience, making them vulnerable to irritable bowel syndrome and exacerbations during times of emotional distress.

A second clinical implication of the amygdala-implant model is its potential relevance to posttraumatic stress disorders (PTSD). These disorders follow after prolonged or repeated exposure to severe, life-threatening stress, such as military combat or violent sexual trauma. Patients manifest sleep disturbances, psychological distress, and enhanced startle reactivity and often engage in heavy alcohol and drug intake. The epidemiology of the disease shows that in combat situations there is a positive dose-response relationship between days of combat exposure and prevalence of the disorder (Bremner et al., 1995). This suggests that some persons are more susceptible than others but that even in the less susceptible, enough exposure to life-threatening circumstances may cause the disorder to appear. The susceptibility hypothesis has been hard to test because volunteers have often been traumatized months or years before being studied. The amygdala-implant model provides avenues for testing PTSD analogues in animals. Most importantly, it suggests that human PTSD symptoms could be caused by a sensitization of the central CRF system following high levels of cortisol exposure at the amygdala. This sensitization would have the effect of shifting the balance between activational or feed-forward processes and negative feedback processes, leading to a permanent shift toward a more reactive HPAC accompanied by frontal-limbic alterations associated with anxiety.

There is a second connection between PTSD, cortisol regulation, and the limbic system. Patients with PTSD have reduced hippocampal volumes, based on neuroimaging studies (Gilbertson et al., 2002). The hippocampus, as we have already noted, is the primary site of negative feedback for cortisol regulation. In general, persons with smaller hippocampal volumes tend to have poorer diurnal regulation of cortisol production. Their diurnal cycle is flatter, showing less shutdown in the evening, and this leads to greater total production of cortisol in a given day. Also, the hippocampus is the only known central nervous system area that spontaneously produces new nerve cells throughout life. New cells are constantly produced in the dentate gyrus, the part of the hippocampus with the greatest exposure to cortisol carried in the cerebrospinal fluid of the temporal lobe's lateral ventricle. Bruce McEwen and Robert Sapolsky have noted that high levels of cortisol exposure can inhibit growth of new cells in the dentate gyrus and can make existing cells more vulnerable to cell death (McEwen & Sapolsky, 1995; Sapolsky, 1996). In an imaging study by Gilbertson et al. (2002) comparing identical twins exposed and not exposed to combat, a small hippocampus was found to be a risk factor for PTSD and not a consequence. If so, such persons may have been vulnerable to traumatic stress effects by being unable to rapidly regulate their stress responses to severe threat, therefore exposing the amygdala to higher cortisol levels and risking an upregulation of amygdala function following the stress of combat. Secondarily, the already smaller amygdala of such patients would be at greater risk due to higher levels of cortisol and greater activation of cortisol during periods of stress.

The topics just discussed suggest that stress cortisol secretion is important not only for regulating the response to stress. High levels of cortisol sensitize the amygdala and its points of communication with the central CRF system. This apparently deleterious response to high levels of stress cortisol secretion may in fact have an adaptive purpose. Mary Dallman et al. (2003), who are responsible for much of the research on cortisol feedback and its regulatory dynamics, argue that this sensitization mechanism allows the HPAC to continue to be responsive even when it has been exposed to high levels of stress and its attendant secretion of cortisol. Secondarily, the exposure of the CNS to high levels of cortisol would indicate that the animal in question might be living in a dangerous environment, in which case hypervigilance and an active stress response might be adaptive, if costly, traits. This sensitization mechanism can therefore be adaptive for a dangerous environment, such as that faced by soldiers in combat. Finally, this work suggests that a biological vulnerability, in the form of a smaller hippocampus, may increase responses to severe stress by providing weaker negative feedback signals to the HPAC.

The Hypothalamic-Sympatho-Adrenomedullary Axis

The other limb of the stress endocrine system is the hypothalamic-sympatho-adrenomedullary axis, which regulates the stress hormone epinephrine. During states of fight-or-flight, the hypothalamus and brainstem send patterned activational signals to the adrenal medulla, whose cells release stored epinephrine into the circulation. This promotes rapid changes in all tissues supplied with beta-adrenoreceptors, as described in Chapter 4. The collective effect of circulating epinephrine's actions is to greatly stimulate the actions and responsivity of all components of the fight-or-flight response, including release of fuel stores from adipose tissue and the liver, increased cardiac output and rate of respiration, dilation of peripheral blood vessels, and enhancement of skeletal muscle contraction.

In relation to our present emphasis on central integrations of the stress response, the secretion of epinephrine is linked to the secretion of cortisol in several ways and at different levels in the system. First, the central CRF system acting on the PVN of the hypothalamus results in CRF output to the pituitary and HPAC activation, simultaneous with PVN neuronal projections activating the sympathetic outputs that project to the adrenal medulla, leading to epinephrine release. Second, the adrenal gland contains both of the secretory tissues of interest: The medulla contains epinephrine, and the cortex secretes cortisol. Third, epinephrine increases ACTH secretion by the pituitary, thus further coordinating the actions of these two limbs of the stress endocrine response during fight-or-flight. Fourth, epinephrine does not regulate its own secretion in the way that cortisol does because it does not pass the blood-brain barrier. Instead, it is regulated indirectly by autonomic reflexes and by cortisol feedback to the PVN, with consequently reduced activation of brainstem sympathetic control centers. These relationships between the HPAC and the sympathoadrenal axis indicate further the extent of the integration between these two limbs of the acute stress response. As we will discuss below with regard to emotional memory, epinephrine and cortisol both play important roles in establishing memories of events having high motivational significance.

Amygdala and Hippocampal Responses to Stress Hormone Feedback: Modulation of Emotional Memory Formation and Working Memory

The presence of receptors for cortisol in the hippocampus, a structure firmly associated with memory, suggests a functional association between brain systems involved with cognitive processes and those associated with the emotions and stress responses. At least part of this emotion-cognition connection operates in the context of stress responses, and perhaps most importantly, because cognitions form the beginning of our formulation of psychological stress responses, we might well imagine that stress-related changes in cognition and memory could have a long-term influence on stress reactivity and psychological and physical well-being.

Most persons are anecdotally aware that emotionally arousing events tend to have a special vividness for them. Anyone old enough remembers where they were and what they were doing when president John Kennedy was shot in 1963. I was a sophomore in high school when a teacher ran into our classroom and turned on the TV set so we could watch the first reports coming from Dallas. The pioneering work by James McGaugh and colleagues (McGaugh & Roozendaal, 2002; Roozendaal, Nguyen, Power, & McGaugh, 1999) has shown us that consolidation for such memories is strongly determined by two stress hormones acting in concert. Epinephrine provides strong feedback to the central nervous system by acting on beta-receptors on the vagus nerve. Vagal inputs to the nucleus of the solitary tract appear to act at the basolateral amygdala to increase its level of activity. This activation in turn acts at the hippocampus and higher centers for memory consolidation to improve retention, and blocking this pathway reduces later recall. During stressful experiences in daily life, cortisol feedback to both the amygdala and hippocampus can be activational, with consequences for formation of declarative memories.

One difficulty in studying the effects of stress on memory in humans is that stress itself has both feed-forward and feedback processes, as discussed above. To begin to disentangle the joint effects of these two sets of events, we performed a study that looked at cortisol feedback to the central nervous system in the absence of the feed-forward processes that accompany stress itself (Buchanan & Lovallo, 2001). To do so, we had subjects visit the lab and take a capsule that contained either a placebo or hydrocortisone (a drug identical to human cortisol). To make this relevant to stress responses, the dose was specifically chosen to raise cortisol levels to match those seen when subjects are stressed in the laboratory. One hour later, the subjects saw a series of emotionally negative, positive, or neutral photographs during a startle modulation procedure. This tests the effect of an emotional or neutral photo on the strength of the startle response to a brief noise burst. We found that cortisol evenly dampened the startle reflex to all types of photographs. Without being told about the memory portion of the study, subjects returned to the lab a week later and were tested on the pictures they had seen. In one test, called cued recall, they were prompted with instructions such as "Tell us all the pictures you can remember that were of accident victims." In this cued recall task, the subjects who had received the stress levels of cortisol at the time of the original task recalled more emotionally relevant material, both positive and negative, but memory for the neutral pictures was the same as under the placebo condition. This study directs attention both to the effects of cortisol on the central nervous system and to the level of emotional activation associated with the pictures as determinants of memory storage. Although more work is needed to fully clarify the mechanisms involved, cortisol feedbacks to the amygdala and hippocampus are reasonable candidates for the site of the memory enhancement. In turn, memory enhancement by cortisol feedback during times of stress would reasonably affect appraisals of future encounters with the same or a similar event (Abercrombie, Kalin, Thurow, Rosenkranz, & Davidson, 2003).

Although cortisol appears to aid in consolidation of long-term memory, it may have the opposite effect on working memory. A dramatic example of the effects of stress on information processing and decision making comes from a visual misclassification by a highly stressed radar operator that had disastrous consequences. On July 3, 1988, the guided missile cruiser *Vincennes* was on patrol in the Persian Gulf at a time of high tension between the United States and the government of Iran. The radar operator reported to the bridge that he saw on his scope a target that was in a "threatening flight profile" (Halloran, 1988) moving toward the ship and descending at an increasing speed—a clear attack signature. After minutes of repeated reports of the aircraft's continued approach, the captain ordered the launch of two surface-to-air missiles. The target was destroyed and was soon identified as Iran Air Flight 655 taking off with a full load of passengers for Dubai. A Pentagon investigation later identified "crew errors" caused by "combat stress" leading to "unconscious distortion of data" (Burns, 1988, pp. 1, 2). Review of the tapes of the communication with the bridge and the time-synchronized radar images showed that during the 5 minutes prior to the missile launch, the operator repeatedly described seeing a descending target and reported a transponder signal consistent with an Iranian F-14 attack jet. Review of the radar images showed a signal indicating an ascending target, and no clear transponder signal was detected. The operator, during a period of emotional stress, had turned his visual inputs upside down and misinterpreted the transponder readings, resulting in 290 deaths.

This interference with working memory may well be related to the short-term effects of stress endocrine feedback to the amygdala and to the prefrontal cortex via amygdaloid outputs to areas in the prefrontal cortex. In our own work, we have often used mental arithmetic as a stressor, and we have incidentally observed that persons with the highest cortisol secretion also have the worst performance on that task, making more mistakes and completing fewer problems (al'Absi, Hugdahl, & Lovallo, 2002; al'Absi et al., 1994). In one such study, we stressed persons with

30 minutes of alternating work on mental arithmetic and a public speaking simulation. As expected, cortisol increased to these two stressors, but more for some persons and less for others. We then had our volunteers work on a different working memory task 30 minutes after the end of the stress portion of the protocol. In this case, we asked them to perform a dichotic listening task. In dichotic listening, the subject hears different syllables (*ba, ka, da,* etc.) presented simultaneously to both ears and reports which syllable, if any, he or she has heard. This is a working memory task in which the subject has to direct attention to auditory inputs, filter out distracting thoughts, and compare inputs with a limited set of six possible syllables. In one version of the task, we instructed subjects to attend to only the right ear. This is easy because the language-dominant left hemisphere processes verbal inputs to the right ear preferentially. Not surprisingly, all subjects did well on this condition. We then asked them to attend to only the left ear and report what they heard. This is much more difficult, and persons typically find it challenging to ignore the dominant right ear inputs. Here the subjects who earlier had produced high levels of cortisol to the stressors were less able to consciously redirect their attention to syllables arriving at the nondominant right hemisphere. Instead, they continued to report more syllables arriving via the right ear and processed in the left hemisphere. This deficit of working memory appeared to be associated with the earlier high levels of cortisol secretion during stress. Work of this sort calls attention to the possible effects of stress on the ability of persons to perform calmly and rationally when required to do so, and it may have implications for knowing who can perform best under highly demanding conditions.

Stress Endocrine Secretion and Regulation of Long-Term Stress Reactivity

The sections above have covered three broad examples of how stress endocrine feedback can alter adaptive behavior. In the first example, we described altered gene expression in the central CRF system and its ability to make the individual more responsive to signals that may indicate danger. This may be adaptive in some circumstances and maladaptive in others. In either case, the effects can be relatively permanent, as in the case of PTSD, resulting in long-term changes in how events are perceived and responded to. The second example, involving formation of long-term, declarative memory, indicates that perceptions and evaluations of ongoing events may be altered for the life of the individual, with consequences for how stress reactions are produced and in relation to which circumstances.

Finally, the combination of amygdaloid sensitization and loss of hippocampal volume could permanently alter not only the individual's cognitive processes but also health more generally. The work of Bruce McEwen and colleagues on the hippocampus and Mary Dallman and colleagues on fuel homeostasis suggests that the effects of stress endocrine feedback, when large and prolonged, may alter the ability of the system to regulate its own cortisol secretion, affecting energy balance and overall health. Studies such as those of Shepard et al. (2000, 2003) on the effects of corticosterone in rats and the related work of Beverley Greenwood-Van Meerveld and colleagues on corticosterone sensitization of pain mechanisms in irritable bowel models suggest that stress levels of glucocorticoid feedback may have relatively direct effects on physical health. These considerations lead us toward a larger synthesis of the effects of stress on homeostasis, with an integration of themes raised in this chapter and in previous ones.

Hierarchy of Autonomic and Endocrine Controls Over Homeostasis

Chapter 5 discussed the functional organization of the organs innervated by the autonomic nervous system. We noted that the entire system was characterized by functional autonomy on the part of individual organs and by modulatory influences and integration of function imposed by higher levels in the system, including the spinal cord, brainstem autonomic nuclei, and the hypothalamus. We can now see that this functional organization also includes the limbic system and the cortex. Most autonomic and endocrine adaptations are functionally complete at the level of the hypothalamus. Reflex organization at this level permits full regulation of organic function and allows the system to respond in an appropriately coordinated fashion to departures from homeostasis.

However, if the system included only the hypothalamus and lower structures, the organism would lack the ability to make behavioral responses, such as finding food, or to respond to distant or future threats. The recognition of an aggressor requires that the aggressor be seen, felt, smelled, or heard. Prior encounters with a threat are useful for preparing us for future encounters. Such functions are the province of a sensory apparatus and a memory system, both associated with the cortex, and with specialized structures for interpreting these events and beginning to formulate a response. We noted that the limbic system, acting through the amygdala, is able to take command of the autonomic and endocrine control centers of the hypothalamus and brainstem when a threat is encountered. This temporarily redirects them from their metabolic and homeostatic chores in order to devote their resources to supporting the behaviors needed to meet the emergency. Thus, the cortex and limbic system represent the highest levels of control in the nervous system, able to supersede, if only briefly, the usual physiological business of maintaining homeostasis.

On the basis of this analysis, we can see that homeostasis is served by an elaborate hierarchy of controls, from intrinsic organ regulation, through the brainstem and hypothalamus, to cortical and limbic areas, and through them to behavior. Felten et al. (1991) have argued that behaviors that restore homeostasis are rewarded, presumably by alteration of limbic system activity. This again argues for a strong linkage between emotions, behavior, and control over our internal states. We noted above that during psychological stress, coping behaviors, whether problem focused or emotion focused, work to reduce the emotional agitation associated with limbic activity. This reduction appears to act as a reward, so long-term behavioral tendencies can act to contribute to the improved maintenance of homeostasis.

The Formation of Psychological Stress Responses Revisited

In this chapter and the two previous ones, we have described the mechanisms by which the brain organizes responses to meet homeostatic demands during stressful events. In previous chapters, we described the peripheral systems active in homeostasis and their expression of the response to some stressors. We also distinguished between physical and psychological stressors, and we indicated that responses to physical stressors, such as exercise, were also engaged during exposure to psychological stressors. In this chapter, we have given a more refined description of psychological stressors as involving cognitive or conditioned appraisals of the threat value of events and appraisals of the outcome of coping responses.

The critical juncture in understanding mechanisms of psychological stress is how primary and secondary appraisals can come to be translated into physical events that influence the state of the body. We have given a partial answer here to our question about the relationship between psychological and physiological events. The frontal lobes, the site of working memory, interact with critical structures in the limbic system and respond in relation to prior experience with certain classes of events. Events that are known or presumed threats are experienced in a way that generates negative emotional responses associated with patterns of interaction among the prefrontal cortex, the amygdala, the hippocampus, and the actions of frontal-limbic areas, including the anterior cingulate gyrus, ventromedial prefrontal cortex, and nucleus accumbens.

The central nucleus of the amygdala, addressing the bed nucleus of the stria terminalis with outputs to the HACER and the PVN of the hypothalamus, is seen as the primary output pathway from these rostral decision-making and evaluative processes and in the development of adaptive neuroendocrine and autonomic responses. The central feedback subsystem defined in Chapter 6 is seen as activating a widespread system of peptide-containing neurons, the central nervous system's CRF system. This system binds together the functions of the cortex, brainstem, and hypothalamus, in turn causing integrated outflow to the periphery.

All the regulatory systems described here can come under the control of events that have primarily symbolic threat value, acting as psychological stressors, and that can be internally generated. Further, these systems designed to maintain homeostasis are ultimately regulated by behavior and in turn shape behaviors according to the behavior's ability to reduce limbic activity associated with distress. So far, we have considered how our perceptions of the world and our perceptions of our ability to cope with challenges in our environment can become the basis for emotional states. Through a process of primary and secondary appraisals, we begin to formulate our physiological responses to psychologically stressful events. Chapter 5 described the layers of control we can use to maintain physiological homeostasis. We now see that we can use our higher cognitive functions, involving frontal areas of the cerebral cortex, to evaluate external events in conjunction with critical structures of the limbic system. These evaluative processes form the basis for emotions and also for the formulation of behavioral, autonomic, and endocrine responses to threatening events. We may therefore think of these psychological processes as exerting the highest level of control over our homeostatic functions. More generally, we may think of the appraisal process and its effects on stress responses as central to our basic question of how ideas can come to have power over our bodies.

Further Reading

Buijs, R. M. (2003). The biological clock tunes the organs of the body: Timing by hormones and the autonomic nervous system. *Journal of Endocrinology, 177,* 17–26.

A concise review of the ability of the paraventricular nucleus to entrain the activity of the peripheral organs in line with light-dark cycles.

Dallman, M. F. (1993). Adaptation of the hypothalamic-pituitary-adrenal axis to chronic stress. *Trends in Endocrinology and Metabolism, 4,* 62–69.

A good review of the primary mechanisms of stress cortisol feedback.

Dallman, M. F., Pecoraro, N., Akana, S. F., La Fleur, S. E., Gomez, F., Houshyar, H., et al. (2003). Chronic stress and obesity: A new view of "comfort food." *Proceedings of the National Academy of Sciences USA, 100*(20), 11696–11701.

This presents a new hypothesis on the mechanisms of stress, cortisol feedback to the central nervous system, and the development of eating disorders.

Greenwood-Van Meerveld, B., Gibson, M., Gunter, W., Shepard, J., Foreman, R., & Myers, D. (2001). Stereotaxic delivery of corticosterone to the amygdala modulates colonic sensitivity in rats. *Brain Research, 893,* 135–142.

New work on the effect of amygdala sensitization by glucocorticoids and its impact on visceral sensitivity, with implications for human irritable bowel syndrome.

McEwen, B. S. (2002). The neurobiology and neuroendocrinology of stress: Implications for post-traumatic stress disorder from a basic science perspective. *Psychiatry Clinics of North America, 25,* 469–494.

A good review of McEwen's model of PTSD and its development following traumatic stress.

McEwen, B. S., & Stellar, E. (1993). Stress and the individual: Mechanisms leading to disease. *Archives of Internal Medicine, 153,* 2093–2101.

A broader work indicating how stress mechanisms may affect health generally.

McGaugh, J. L., & Roozendaal, B. (2002). Role of adrenal stress hormones in forming lasting memories in the brain. *Current Opinion in Neurobiology, 12,* 205–210.

This presents a concise review of the current status of work on stress hormones and memory.

Sapolsky, R. M., Krey, L. C., & McEwen, B. S. (1985). Prolonged glucocorticoid exposure reduces hippocampal neuron number: Implications for aging. *Journal of Neuroscience, 5,* 1222–1227.

A focus on the loss of hippocampal neurons and the potential impact of such loss on glucocorticoid regulation and health.

Shepard, J. D., Barron, K. W., & Myers, D. A. (2000). Corticosterone delivery to the amygdala increases corticotropin-releasing factor mRNA in the central amygdaloid nucleus and anxiety-like behavior. *Brain Research, 861,* 288–295.

A demonstration of a new model of how stress levels of glucocorticoid hormones may sensitize the amygdala to subsequent exposure to anxiety-provoking stimuli.

8

The Immune
System and Behavior

S ince Selye's (1936) earliest work, we have known that high levels
of cortisol occurring during states of stress can alter immune system
tissues and suppress immune system responses. This led to the insight
that mechanisms serving the response to a stressor have an impact on
immune system function. At the same time, Selye saw infection itself as a
stressor because it threatens the organism and causes both nonspecific
and specific compensatory responses. Both observations suggested that
immune responses and generalized stress responses interact with each
other. Since then, our recognition of the interactions between immune
function and autonomic and endocrine mechanisms has grown substantially. In this chapter, we will briefly describe the organization of the
immune response and then provide some examples of interplay between
immune function and stress-related autonomic and endocrine responses.
We will see that higher cortical and limbic integrations ultimately modulate immune responses just as they control autonomic and endocrine
responses.

Overview of the Immune System

Vertebrate organisms have evolved the capacity to detect and attack
harmful invaders or their own cells when these have become abnormal
and have the potential to do harm. Foreign organisms include bacteria,

viruses, fungi, and parasites. Altered endogenous cells are those that are transformed by malignancy or infected by a virus. Immunologists refer to these collectively as *antigen*.

To aid in survival, the immune system recognizes antigen, neutralizes it, and then remembers specific antigen for future reference. So the immune system has the ability to perceive, respond to, and remember antigen. These are functions we usually associate with the central nervous system, and the recognition of these cognitivelike capacities in a set of non-neuronal cells residing in the body is quite striking. The immune system has been referred to as a "mobile surveillance system" (J. F. Sheridan, personal communication, August 1995) and a "circulating brain" (E. M. Sternberg, personal communication, August 1995). A thorough discussion of the immune system is provided by Kuby (1994).

The immune system is composed of a set of structural components, including organs, tissues, and cells, whose activity is coordinated by a set of messenger substances. These structural components, in conjunction with immune messengers, have both innate functions and functions acquired by experience.

Structural Components of the Immune System

The structural components of the immune system are *barriers* to infection, including skin and mucous membranes; the *immune cells* that actually contact antigens and neutralize them; and the *immune organs* and *tissues* that produce and support the immune system cells.

Immune System Organs and Tissues

The tissues of the immune system include the bone marrow, thymus, lymph nodes, and spleen. Collectively, these are known as *lymphoid tissues* and are sites of production, maturation, and activation of immune system cells. The bone marrow generates the immature, undifferentiated stem cells that develop into the specialized cells that act on antigen. B cells mature in the bone marrow before entering the circulation and traveling to lymph nodes and the spleen. T cells mature in the thymus, an organ located above the heart, before entering the circulation and traveling also to lymph nodes and the spleen. These latter two lymphoid organs trap antigen and provide a place for activation of T and B cells by contact with the trapped antigen.

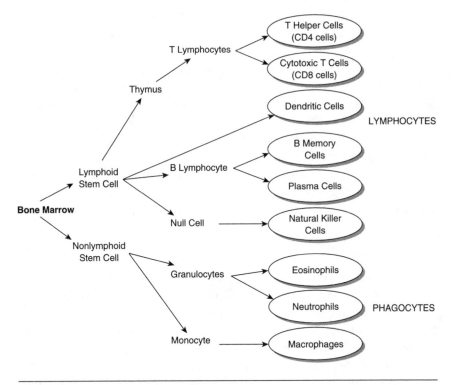

Figure 8.1   Origins of immune system cells. All immune system cells are derived ultimately from the stem cells found in bone marrow.

Immune System Cells

The immune system cells are all specialized, differentiated forms of white blood cells originally derived from stem cells of the bone marrow. They spend part of their time in circulation and part in the lymphatic system, thymus, and spleen. There are two major classes of immune system cells: *phagocytes* and *lymphocytes*. As can be seen in Figure 8.1, these develop through one or more stages before reaching their mature forms and becoming capable of acting as immune cells.

Phagocytes

As their name implies, phagocytes ingest and destroy antigen. Phagocytes mature from nonlymphoid stem cells and form two classes, *monocytes* and *granulocytes*. The monocytes produce macrophages, whereas the granulocytes generate both neutrophils and eosinophils.

Although the three types of phagocytes differ in their modes of killing, they all migrate to sites of infection, being attracted by local chemical messengers, where they ingest antigen.

Macrophages are noteworthy among the phagocytes because they play a key role in triggering a full immune response. After breaking down antigen, macrophages attach antigen fragments to a specialized protein, known as the *major histocompatibility complex* (MHC). They then express the antigen-MHC complex on their surfaces and present the complex to maturing T cells. This stimulates development of T helper cells and results in production of a family of messengers called *cytokines*. The macrophages themselves are also active secretors of cytokines that further help to stimulate and coordinate the immune response.

Lymphocytes

The *lymphocytes* consist of T cells, B cells, and natural killer (NK) cells.

NK cells act as an innate cellular surveillance team to slow the development of antigen, thereby allowing time for other immune mechanisms to come into play. NK cells are genetically programmed to recognize tumor cells and virally infected cells. Using our cognitive analogy, we might call this genetic endowment of disease-recognizing cells a very long-term memory system by which our species has learned which microorganisms are dangerous and how to destroy them.

The *B lymphocytes* have antigen-binding proteins called *antibodies* on their surfaces. Antibodies are immunoglobulins, one class of globulin proteins found in the blood. In the surveillance process, B cells trap antigen on the antibodies and then internalize and process the antigen and present fragments on their surface MHC to the T cells. This B cell–to–T cell contact stimulates division and multiplication of B cells into *plasma cells* and *B memory cells*. Plasma cells and B memory cells then produce antibody specific to the antigen that originally triggered their development. Plasma cells then secrete large numbers of free antibodies that circulate in the bloodstream for the duration of a disease. These circulating free antibodies inactivate free antigen found in the blood before they invade the cells of the body. Their companions, the B memory cells, live on indefinitely following contact with a novel antigen and continue to express specific antibodies on their surfaces. It is these antibodies that are later found in circulation following vaccination or an episode of infection.

The *T lymphocytes* mature in the thymus, where they become either *T helper cells* or *cytotoxic T cells*. All T cells carry antigen-recognizing molecules known as T-cell receptors.

T helper cells form the focal point of the response to invasion by exogenous antigen such as virus particles, bacteria, or fungi. Exogenous antigen is presented to T helper cells on the surface MHC of macrophages or B cells. The T helper cell has an auxiliary surface molecule, known as CD4, that assists the T-cell receptor to respond to the presented antigen. In response, T helper cells secrete cytokines to activate B cells, cytotoxic T cells, macrophages, and NK cells. The progressive loss of CD4 cells during infection with human immunodeficiency virus (HIV) is the reason that this disease ultimately eliminates the immune response to infection. As a result, most deaths due to HIV are from opportunistic infections by other agents.

Dendritic cells are poorly understood. They derive from bone marrow cells and appear in lymph nodes and other organs of the immune system. They attach to antigen using their dendritic processes and present antigen on MHC-II receptors. They appear to be able to activate cytotoxic T cells.

The cytotoxic T cells possess a different auxiliary surface receptor, known as CD8. They can respond to antigen-presenting cells such as dendritic cells, and they are highly responsive to endogenous cells that are virally infected or tumor altered. Therefore, these cells are specialized for killing the body's own cells that have become tumor cells or have been infected by a virus.

Immune System Messengers

The development, maturation, and activity of immune system cells are coordinated by a set of messengers known collectively as *cytokines* (for *cell-acting* substances). Cytokines are produced by immune system cells or by infected cells, and in turn they affect the function of distant tissues, nearby cells, and the very cells that secrete them. Table 8.1 indicates some of the principal cytokines and their actions. In orchestrating the immune response, the most important sources of cytokines are macrophages and T helper cells. Their cytokines (a) stimulate immune cell replication and division by altering gene expression; (b) stimulate immune cells to neutralize antigen and to secrete other cytokines; (c) cause B cells to form antibodies; and (d) help immune cells to recognize the antigen in the future.

Because of their signaling role, cytokines can generate interactions of the immune system with behavior. At the hypothalamus, cytokines induce illness-related behaviors including sleep, reduced movement, and loss of appetite and sexual function. Cytokines also induce nonspecific

Table 8.1   Some Principal Cytokines and Their Actions

Cytokine	Source	Actions
Interleukin-1	Macrophages B cells	Maturation and development of B cells. Activation of T cells.
Interleukin-2	T helpers	Proliferation and development of NK cells.
Interleukin-4	T helpers	Activation and proliferation of B cells. Phagocyte growth and proliferation.
Interleukin-6	Macrophages T helpers	Inflammation at site of infection, plasma cell information. Hypothalamic activation.
Interleukin-10	T helpers	Macrophage activation.
Interferon-gamma	T helpers	B-cell activation, macrophage.

endocrine responses via the pituitary-adrenal axis, especially secretion of stress levels of cortisol.

Having briefly considered the structure of the immune system, its cells, and the cytokines, we will consider how these act in concert during an infection. The two functional components of the immune system are *innate resistance* and *acquired resistance*.

Innate Resistance

Each of us is born with an innate immune capability. The body's innate resistance encompasses (a) structural defenses; (b) locally produced chemical signals that an infection is in progress; (c) innate cellular responses; and (d) nonspecific neuroendocrine-immune interactions.

Our *structural defenses,* including skin and the lining of the mouth and gut, are positioned as a first line of defense to resist invasion of the body by pathogens. However, foreign organisms that manage to find their way into the blood or other tissues must then be removed by specific mechanisms.

The presence of antigen in local tissues causes release of specialized *chemical signals* that attract macrophages and the other phagocytes to the site of infection, where they ingest antigen. Subsets of B cells and T cells are programmed to begin the *innate cellular response* to an infection. At birth, we have a small, innate population of reactive T cells that immediately becomes activated by our first infection and is continually modified by future antigen encounters. We are also born with a large number of genetically determined B-cell antibodies. These genetically determined antibodies have been shaped by selection over generations of experience with various pathogens.

The fourth component of our natural immune response is nonspecific *neuroendocrine–immune system* interactions. These involve cytokine-mediated secretion of epinephrine and cortisol, which in turn act as nonspecific global regulators of the immune response (Scheinman, Cogswell, Lofquist, & Baldwin, 1995).

Acquired Resistance and Establishment of Immune System Memory

Soon after birth, through repeated antigen exposure, our immune system matures and develops its own unique complement of antibodies and a population of specialized T cells and B memory cells. Using our earlier metaphor of the immune system as a circulating brain, we might say that the maturing immune system has learned from experience and memorized a list of antigen that it has previously seen. It has also developed adaptive responses to that list of antigen. As a result, the immune response has become more rapid and precisely focused.

A mature immune response has three phases. During the *inductive phase,* macrophages and T helper cells respond to antigen with specific cellular and cytokine responses. During the *effector phase,* mediators in lymphoid tissue take over to produce antibodies and lethal immune cells, and these activated immune cells travel to the site of an infection and destroy antigen. This results in a set of *functional immune changes* able to respond rapidly to later contact with the same antigen. These stages are diagrammed in Figure 8.2.

The Inductive Phase

During the inductive phase, (a) bacteria or virus particles attract *macrophages* and *B cells,* or (b) tumor-altered cells or virally altered cells attract *macrophages* and *NK cells.* Macrophages ingest antigen and begin secreting the cytokines interleukin-1 (IL-1) and IL-6, resulting in the effects listed in Table 8.1. Also, macrophages process the antigen for presentation

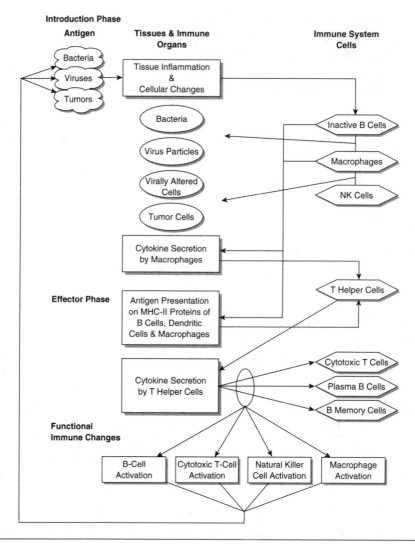

Figure 8.2 Stages of the immune response to invasion by antigen. The immune response proceeds in three stages: induction phase, effector phase, and functional immune changes. Each phase is associated with a different complement of immune system cells engaged in different forms of activity and being in different functional states. The *induction phase* begins when an invasion by antigen causes inflammation and other changes in local tissues. These result in release of cytokine messengers and cellular attractants that cause an initial response by immune system cells prepared to react to these early signals. In the *effector phase*, cytokines and antigen presentation by B cells, macrophages, and dendritic cells are shown activating T helper cells. These key immune system cells in turn stimulate the mature immune response by cytotoxic T cells, plasma cells, and B memory cells, causing the full spectrum of functional immune changes. These *functional immune changes* are collectively able to rid the body of antigen, and they close the loop on the immune response.

on MHC to T helper cells. This causes T helper cells to stimulate themselves by secreting IL-2, to become *activated T helper cells.*

T helper cell activation is the central step in the induction of the immune response because T helper cell cytokines then trigger development of specific activated T- and B-cell populations. The achievement of a fully developed immune response can take up to 7 days, the length of time we usually take to begin to recover from a common cold. The T helper cell is consequently the single most important element in the immune system. It has the characteristics to allow it to generate a broad range of specific cytokines to fine-tune the development of the effector phase of the immune response.

The Effector Phase

During the effector phase of the immune response, T helper cell cytokines stimulate both major branches of the specific immune response: (a) T cells mature into cytotoxic T cells, responsible for *cell-mediated immunity;* and (b) B lymphocytes mature into plasma cells, responsible for *humoral immunity.* Cytokines also activate NK cells and macrophages.

In cell-mediated immunity, inactive cytotoxic T cells are stimulated by cytokines to become activated cytotoxic T lymphocytes able to destroy cells that have been altered by viral invasion or carcinogenic processes. In humoral immunity, B cells, performing their antigen surveillance role in the circulation or in lymph nodes, come in contact with antigen and present it to T helper cells already activated by IL-2. This causes the activated T helper cells to secrete IL-2, IL-4, IL-6, and interferon-gamma. The B cells then differentiate and multiply to become either B memory cells or plasma cells. The plasma cells travel to lymph nodes, the spleen, and the sites of active infection and begin producing large quantities of free antibody that enter circulation. These circulating free-antibody particles can surround and inactivate antigen. The steps are summarized in the middle portion of Figure 8.2.

To briefly summarize the effector phase, antigen presentation to T helper cells and their resultant IL-2 secretion result in production of cell-killing cytotoxic T lymphocytes, antibody production by plasma cells, and the production of B memory cells. These resultant cells are shown in the lower right portion of Figure 8.2.

Functional Immune Changes

The inductive phase also results in the production of long-lived T memory cells and the B memory cells that carry specific antibodies. At this stage, the full immune response cycle has been completed, and the system is primed to ward off future attacks by the same antigen.

The Behavior-Immune Interface

We said at the beginning of this chapter that Selye's work suggested an interaction between immune function and stress responses. In fact, there are four points of contact: (a) The immune system signals the central nervous system with cytokines; (b) the central nervous system regulates the immune response through the pituitary-adrenocortical axis; (c) immune system cells have receptors for epinephrine; and (d) the organs of the immune system are innervated by both branches of the autonomic nervous system (Felten & Felten, 1991). This two-way communication opens many possibilities for considering the behavioral interactions with the immune system.

Immune-to-Behavior Communication

In discussing cytokines, we noted that some of these are able to reach the hypothalamus, where they induce secretion of stress levels of cortisol and also produce what immunologists call *illness behaviors*. In animal studies, injection of IL-1 or IL-6 either systemically or into the third ventricle, adjacent to the hypothalamus, leads to a full range of illness behaviors. The hypothalamus has numerous cytokine receptors, suggesting a specific signaling role to this important regulatory area. We are all familiar with the powerful feeling of being sick. This malaise is a nonspecific response: It has similar characteristics regardless of the specific illness we may have. At the beginning, we may notice nothing more than a vague mood disturbance, a feeling of impatience and irritability. Soon we begin to feel that all is not well, and gradually we recognize that we are sick. Shortly after, we find ourselves wanting to withdraw from activities, to become inactive, and to sleep if possible. At the same time, we lose our appetite for food and our interest in pleasurable activities such as listening to music, seeing a movie, or engaging in sex.

The generation of illness behaviors is paralleled by activation of stress levels of corticotropin releasing factor (CRF) via the magnocellular portion of the paraventricular nucleus of the hypothalamus. This activation of the stress-related part of the CRF system results in secretion of high levels of cortisol, involving alterations in mood and causing other changes within the central nervous system.

Behavior-to-Immune Communication

If we recognize that components of stress responses can alter the immune system, then we have an important key for thinking about one way immune function can be altered by behavior. We have discussed in previous chapters how emotions and cognitions can alter activity in important limbic structures, including the hippocampus and amygdala. These in turn can signal the hypothalamus to modify both hormonal secretions via the adrenal gland and sympathetic outflow by the autonomic nervous system.

The adrenal and sympathetic components of the stress response have pervasive influences on the immune system. Lymphoid tissues including thymus, spleen, and lymph nodes receive inputs from both sympathetic and parasympathetic neurons. Changes in autonomic activity will affect these tissues and alter the development and activity of populations of lymphocytes, including NK, T, and B cells. So the cell populations needed to orchestrate the destruction of invading organisms are directly altered by autonomic activity accompanying emotional activation and stress.

Lymphocytes have beta-adrenoreceptors and glucocorticoid receptors. The effects of catecholamines on lymphocyte receptors can be complex, both increasing and decreasing indicators of immune system function. For example, stimulation of beta-receptors can reduce the ability of NK cells to enter lymph nodes, where they can contact and neutralize antigen (Ottaway & Husband, 1992). At the same time, epinephrine can cause splenic contraction, releasing stored lymphocytes into the general circulation and increasing their ability to travel to sites of infection. Beta-adrenergic activation accompanying acute stress can increase NK cell numbers in circulation and decrease the ability of T cells to multiply to appropriate stimuli (Bachen et al., 1995). This range of effects is a caution against thinking that stress always impairs the immune system. Instead, it is important to consider the specific situations under which enhancements and decreases in function may occur.

The immune system also has important interactions with the hypothalamic-pituitary-adrenocortical axis (HPAC). Stress levels of cortisol can inhibit immune function in several ways, including (a) decreased macrophage expression of MHC in response to IL-2 or interferon-gamma; (b) decreased macrophage cell ingestion; (c) decreased IL-1 production by macrophages; (d) decreased IL-2 production by T cells; (e) decreased production of CD4 cells; (f) suppressed activity of B lymphocytes; and (g) decreased activity of NK cells. These changes amount to a reduction of the frequency and strength of immune system messages and a reduction of the numbers and activity of cells carrying out immune responses. In contrast to sympathetic activity and circulating epinephrine, stress levels of cortisol may well exert largely deleterious effects on immune function. This may call attention to situations and emotional states accompanied by cortisol elevations as being particularly worthy of study as potential impairments to immune function.

The interface between immune function and our emotions and behaviors consists of integrated neural and hormonal messages that allow for communication in both directions. There are several examples of this communication at work, and all invite interesting speculations about the relationship between health and behavior.

Immunologists formerly viewed the immune system as highly autonomous in its actions, responding only to the presence of antigen. They criticized the idea that the stress response could have more than nonspecific effects on immune function. More recent views emphasize that the immune system is modulated by a hierarchy of controls involving the hypothalamus, limbic system, and cerebral cortex (Rozlog, Kiecolt-Glaser, Marucha, Sheridan, & Glaser, 1999). Felten et al. (1991) have suggested that the immune system is ultimately under behavioral control.

Behavior-Immune Interactions and Health Indicators

The interaction of immune system function and stress mechanisms can be illustrated by several examples. The first concerns stress effects on immune system activation to viral challenge and on reactivation of latent viruses. The second has to do with altered risk for arthritis due to deficient cortisol secretion. The third example concerns changes in specific immune system indicators during life stressors.

Stress, Immune Response to Viral Challenge, and Viral Reactivation

Under normal circumstances, infection with an active influenza strain or vaccination with an inactive virus will produce an immune response measurable in the number of antibody particles found in the circulation. However, increases in stress levels and their associated elevations in cortisol and sympathetic nervous system activity can suppress this immune system activation by viral challenges. For example, repeated restraint stress in mice can alter production of antibodies and lower T-cell activation in response to infection with influenza virus (Sheridan & Dobbs, 1994). Restraint stress also reduces the ability of mononuclear cells to respond to viral infection by accumulating in lymph nodes, where they would normally consume virus-infected cells. Blocking the action of corticosterone restores the activity level of these cells in stressed animals (Hermann, Beck, & Sheridan, 1995).

Similar evidence in humans suggests that stress lowers the body's response to viral challenge. In this model, a vaccine is administered to persons who have experienced a naturalistic stressor, and the ability of the immune system to develop antibodies to that vaccine is considered a clinically relevant measure of the integrity of the immune response. Work using this approach has shown that hepatitis B vaccine produces a stronger antibody response in medical students reporting better social support and less global stress (Glaser, Kiecolt-Glaser, Bonneau, Malarkey, & Hughes, 1992). These studies suggest that stress and negative emotional states are likely to lower the immune system's ability to mount a successful response to a challenge with either an active virus or a vaccination. The specific mechanisms of such a behavior-immune interaction are not yet fully identified, although elevated cortisol and sympathetic nervous system activity appear to be mediators.

There appear to be important individual differences in the degree to which stress cortisol activation will suppress the immune response to viral challenge. As we will see in Chapter 10, individuals who have large cardiac sympathetic nervous system responses to stress typically have large cortisol responses to stressors that are anxiety or fear provoking (al'Absi et al., 1997). In a study by Douglas Carroll and colleagues, persons showing the greatest sympathetic and cortisol activation to acute stress in the laboratory were also the ones with the poorest antibody response to a hepatitis B vaccination program (Burns, Ring, Drayson, & Carroll, 2002). Although this study does not address the issue, it suggests that habitual sympathetic and adrenocortical responsivity can be associated with reduced immune system responsivity. The relationship between laboratory stress reactivity and immune system function also extends to natural occurrence of disease.

A closely related research model of immune system function tests persons exposed to stressors in their daily lives and looks for evidence of reactivation of latent viruses such as herpes simplex or Epstein-Barr viruses (Bonneau, 1994). In the case of herpes simplex, after a person has had an initial infection, the viruses become dormant within the cell bodies of the sensory and autonomic neurons innervating the originally infected tissues. They can remain dormant in this way for long periods, and because they are inactive within the cell body, there are no changes on the cell membrane for the immune system to detect. However, as many of us know, emotional distress can trigger reactivation of these latent viruses, as seen in the recurrent outbreak of fever blisters in persons undergoing life stress (Jemmott & Locke, 1984) and, in the case of Epstein-Barr virus, among adolescents who tend to develop mononucleosis when over-worked and underrested. In tests of the effect of stress on viral reactivation, medical students undergoing the stress of examinations were more likely to have outbreaks of herpes if they lacked social support (Glaser, Kiecolt-Glaser, Speicher, & Holliday, 1985). Similarly, exam stress was associated with high levels of antibody to Epstein-Barr virus, suggesting reactivation of latent infections (Glaser et al., 1987). Similar indicators of decreased immune surveillance are seen in men undergoing divorce and experiencing poor marital relationships (Keller, Shiflett, Schliefer, & Bartlett, 1994).

The mechanisms of viral reactivation are not fully understood, although both sympathetic nervous system activity and HPA activation may be involved. Jenkins and Baum (1995) noted that reactivation of her-pes simplex virus is preceded by high levels of nerve growth factor. Nerve growth factor is produced in surrounding tissues in response to sympa-thetic nerve activity. Sympathetic activation, associated with acute stress and negative emotional states, may lead to increases in nerve growth fac-tor, triggering reactivation of latent herpes viruses in affected nerves and target tissues. Viral latency is also maintained by active immune surveil-lance, and suppression of immune function may permit reactivation to occur. The magnitude of cortisol response to acute stressors administered in the laboratory appears to be significantly correlated in several studies with level of antibodies to Epstein-Barr virus, suggesting greater reacti-vation of the virus in the most stress-reactive persons (Cacioppo et al., 2002; Larson, Ader, & Moynihan, 2001). Cortisol is specifically able to stimulate replication of latent virus (Cacioppo et al., 2002; Glaser, Kutz, MacCallum, & Malarkey, 1995). Therefore, cortisol levels high enough to suppress immune function also permit reactivation of herpes viruses. These reactions are likely to be greatest in persons with the highest level of reactivity to psychological stressors.

Altered Rheumatoid Arthritis
Susceptibility and Altered HPAC Function

We have noted that illness is itself a stressor and that peripheral cytokines find their way to the hypothalamus, where they cause the secretion of stress levels of cortisol. What is the adaptive value of the immune system generating stress levels of cortisol that can impair the immune response? The answer seems to be that the immune response works best when regulated. If the immune system is underresponsive, we risk being overwhelmed by invading organisms. But in the absence of regulation, the immune response would run unchecked, with massive quantities of inflammatory cytokines being secreted. Too much inflammation can damage healthy tissue, causing problems above and beyond the effects of the illness itself. One reason we take aspirin when we are sick is to reduce inflammatory responses. For the same reason, we put ice on an injury. The healing is faster and more problem free if the injured tissue does not become too inflamed. High levels of cytokines can even be deadly. In the case of toxic shock syndrome, the victim can die within hours from an unregulated immune response.

During the early phases of an infection, the HPAC produces cortisol in response to cytokines from peripheral infection. Similarly, the hypothalamic-adrenomedullary axis is stimulated to produce epinephrine. The high levels of cortisol production induced by the activation of the HPAC suppress inflammation at the site of infection and control cellular responses by lymphoid tissues. This results in lowered production of immune cells, fewer cytokines, and less inflammation of infected tissues, further reducing cytokine production. This negative feedback relationship between the cytokine signaling system and the HPAC during infection is essential to the proper regulation of the immune response.

The dangers of an unregulated immune system are illustrated by research on the cause of the inflammatory disease rheumatoid arthritis. In this form of arthritis, the joints become chronically inflamed and are swollen and deformed. The disease is crippling, often making it impossible for the victim to work. Women are about four times as likely to develop rheumatoid arthritis as men. Women also have more active immune systems than men do (Morell, 1995). Research into the causes of this debilitating and painful disease has concentrated on two companion strains of inbred rats known as the Lewis and Fischer strains. The story of this odd couple of the rodent world is important because it illustrates how behavioral mechanisms related to the stress response, and acting through the HPAC, can affect mechanisms of disease.

The Lewis rat is highly susceptible to arthritis. Researchers have long known that infecting Lewis rats with streptococcus bacterium ultimately results in arthritis of the paw joints. It seems that in these rats the strep infection runs unchecked and results in the development of severe, chronic joint inflammation. This ultimately leads to joint swelling and deformity, as seen in human sufferers. On the other hand, a close relative of the Lewis rat, the Fischer rat, is highly resistant to arthritis. Attempts to induce persistent inflammation by infecting them with various bacterial strains fail to produce any untoward effects. Eventually, it was discovered that the differing fates of these two rat strains was determined by differences in their HPAC reactivity. It is significant that the Lewis rat is not able to produce a normal corticosterone response to behavioral stress, although the Fischer rat produces a robust response (Moncek, Kvetnansky, & Jezova, 2001).

Esther Sternberg and her colleagues at the National Institute of Mental Health discovered that the Lewis rat is highly deficient in its ability to secrete corticosterone during stress or in response to normal metabolic stimuli (Sternberg et al., 1989). On the other hand, the Fischer rat is a corticosterone hypersecretor—anything likely to cause a rat to secrete corticosterone produces an exaggerated response by these rats. The difference in HPAC reactivity in these rats that differ in disease susceptibility is more than coincidence: The difference in corticosterone secretion underlies the difference in disease proneness.

These rat strains are *histocompatible;* the genes encoding their major histocompatibility complexes are identical, and they can accept tissue donations from each other without danger of rejection. Through a careful series of tissue transplantation experiments, Sternberg et al. determined that the two strains differ in their hypothalamic areas controlling synthesis and secretion of CRF. By transplanting portions of the hypothalamus from the Fischer to the Lewis rat, it is possible to make the Lewis recipient normally resistant to arthritis. Similarly, removing these portions of the hypothalamus from the Fischers makes them as vulnerable to arthritis as the Lewis rats. Apparently, these hypothalamic transplants augment the deficient stress corticosterone secretion in the Lewis rat.

The relationship between deficient HPAC responsiveness and rheumatoid arthritis leads to the speculation that emotions acting through this axis can alter arthritis susceptibility. Sternberg has proposed that deficient HPAC activity accompanying depression may link depression with enhanced susceptibility to, or greater severity of, rheumatoid arthritis (Sternberg, Wilder, Chrousos, & Gold, 1991). Related evidence indicates that low levels of cortisol or reduced cortisol response to infection can result in poor regulation of an inflammatory response with increased mortality. In this case, Wistar rats were exposed to two episodes of social defeat and later inoculated with lipopolysaccharide antigen. The defeated animals had a deficient corticosterone response to this inflammatory challenge, accompanied by higher than normal levels of cytokines and an increased rate of morality (Carobrez, Gasparotto, Buwalda, & Bohus, 2002). This study suggests that the increased inflammatory response that is genetically determined in the Lewis rat may also be induced in other rat strains by life experience, with significant consequences for the socially stressed animal.

Altered Immune Function and Life Stress in Humans

Studies of artificial stressors in the laboratory have many advantages, but they do not readily allow us to study how people are affected by events in their daily lives. However, studies of life stressors and their effects on health and health indicators can give us useful insights into the effects of stress on health. Although a stress-related reduction in vaccine response is a useful experimental model, it can also have significant implications in cases of real-life stress where large-scale vaccination programs may become ineffective during periods when population stress levels are high (Yang & Glaser, 2002). Tests of antibody responses to vaccines given to troops about to invade Kuwait during the Gulf War of 1991 showed lower than expected antibody response rates. High stress among troops about to be sent into combat appears to be a plausible explanation.

One method of studying life stress is to follow persons exposed to natural disasters for their psychological reactions and physical consequences. Such events can result in prolonged feelings of helplessness and psychological distress associated with altered endocrine function and immune system indicators. Andrew Baum and colleagues (Baum, 1990; McKinnon, Weisse, Reynolds, Bowles, & Baum, 1989) examined residents of the area around the Three-Mile Island nuclear plant near Harrisburg, Pennsylvania, following the 1979 radiation leak and emergency reactor shutdown. After the accident, compared to controls, residents felt more psychological distress, had higher urinary catecholamines, and had higher antibodies to herpes simplex virus, and their immune function showed lowered levels of T, B, and NK cells. Residents also had a prolongation of cardiovascular responses to mental arithmetic stress. Years after the accident, some residents had higher blood pressures than before it occurred. These changes indicate a state of chronic stress with depressed immune function and elevated sympathetic nervous system activity.

Other studies of stress in daily life concern the effects of examinations on students and daily stressors in a community sample. Medical students predictably show higher levels of psychological distress and elevated blood pressure, catecholamines, and cortisol on days of major exams (Herbert, Moore, de la Riva, & Watts, 1986; Sausen, Lovallo, Pincomb, & Wilson,

1992). Students report more illness surrounding exam periods and have higher antibodies to Epstein-Barr virus and lower T-cell activation and cytokine secretion (Glaser et al., 1987). In a community sample, reported daily life stress was associated with lowered activation of the immune response to challenge with a novel, harmless antigen (Stone et al., 1994). These show that there may be deficiencies of immune function in relation to the experience of stress in the school setting and possibly the workplace.

Whereas studies such as the above focus on immune system indicators, others have examined actual susceptibility to illness in persons experiencing stressful life events. Kawachi et al. (1995) showed that nurses who had performed rotating shift work for more than 6 years of their working lives had a significantly increased risk of heart disease and heart attack than nurses who had worked normal daytime shifts. Although heart disease is not usually associated with immune system dysregulation, recent models of the atherogenic process give a major role to cytokine production in the affected arteries and to macrophages and other phagocytes in their role as scavengers of damaged cells and lipids in the atherosclerotic lesion. This study provides significant evidence of the deleterious effects of prolonged low levels of stress on health.

Similar evidence comes from a study of the effects of acute infection with cold viruses. Cohen (1994) exposed volunteers to nose drops containing one of several varieties of cold viruses or to a saline solution and followed them for several days to note which ones developed actual colds, had subclinical signs of respiratory changes, or had immune system responses indicating an infection. Volunteers experiencing more negative life events along with poor coping responses and negative emotional states were more likely to have higher rates of infection and to actually contract colds. Negative life events were the strongest predictor of these reactions.

In a study of life stress, stress reactivity, and actual incidence of disease, Cohen et al. (2002) tested lab stress reactivity on two occasions, documented who had the largest cortisol reactions, and then followed subjects for 12 weeks to test for occurrence of illness. Those who had the largest cortisol reactions to stress and who had encountered the largest number of natural stressors, in the form of negative life events, were the ones who had the most upper respiratory infections during the follow-up. The study documented actual occurrence of illness rather than simply relying on self-report. Although the advice may be premature, some have advocated laboratory stress testing as a means to document immune system competence and potential risk for disease (Boone & Anthony, 2003).

Our final example of the effects of emotional stress on immune function comes from the effects of difficult personal relationships. Kiecolt-Glaser and colleagues have conducted a longitudinal study of the psychological and health effects on elderly persons involved in chronic care of a spouse with Alzheimer's disease. Alzheimer's is an untreatable, progressive dementia that severely alters the personality and impairs communication and cognitive capacity. It places a severe burden on spouses who are caregivers. The disease signals a permanent and irreversible change in a loved one and a loss of support within the marriage. Bearing the burden of such a demand constitutes a meaningful, long-term life stressor to the elderly caregiver.

The act of caring for an Alzheimer's patient is time demanding, and caregivers usually have fewer social contacts and less time to spend with the ones they do have. They experience physical and mental fatigue and negative emotions, especially depression. In this study, the spouses who were most distressed by their partner's dementia and who were lowest in social support also showed lowered levels of cellular immunity and had more frequent respiratory tract infections. Among these caregivers, those who had the largest heart rate increases to mental arithmetic stress in the laboratory also had the largest cortisol responses and the greatest alterations in NK cell function to the stressor (Kiecolt-Glaser, Malarkey, Cacioppo, & Glaser, 1994). Compared to age-matched controls, caregivers of Alzheimer patients also show slower healing of superficial wounds to the skin, a process dependent on cytokine production in injured tissue and on the macrophage response to these cytokines (Kiecolt-Glaser, Marucha, Malarkey, Mercado, & Glaser, 1995). This stress-related suppression of wound healing is also seen in more acute forms of life stress, such as exam stress in medical students (Marucha, Kiecolt-Glaser, & Favagehi, 1998). Other work supports a linkage between the chronic stress of caregiving, greater cardiovascular responses to mental stress, enhanced cortisol activation, and immune system modulation (Uchino, Cacioppo, Malarkey, & Glaser, 1995). In addition to slower wound healing, caregivers experience poorer health generally and have more infectious illness than noncaregivers, with a slightly greater impact of caregiving stress appearing in women (Vitaliano, Zhang, & Scanlon, 2003).

Further studies on the wound-healing model in fact suggest that the stress effects are mediated by cortisol activation. Sheridan and colleagues (Padgett, Marucha, & Sheridan, 1998) showed that restraint stress applied before and after experimental skin wounding in mice caused reduced inflammation and prolonged healing. The effect of the stressor was prevented by glucocorticoid receptor blockade, suggesting that the wound-healing effect is mediated by elevated cortisol during exposure to the stressors. In addition to slower wound healing, restraint stress also increases the risk of opportunistic infection of the wound site, further implicating the effects of stress and cortisol activation on reduced immune system function (Rojas, Padgett, Sheridan, & Marucha, 2002).

Stress Buffers, Positive Emotions, and Physical Health

The examples of behavior-immune interactions given above concern the effect of negative emotions and life stress on the immune system. Whether there are parallel enhancements of immune function accompanying positive behavioral states is not currently known. However, the possible buffering effects of positive emotions, positive human relationships, and enhanced feelings of self-efficacy are thought to ameliorate the negative effects of life stress on immune function (Kiecolt-Glaser, McGuire, Robles, & Glaser, 2002). Although there is less research on enhanced immune function in relationship to positive emotions, some suggestive examples from the psychological literature encourage us to think that behavior can be used in positive ways to counteract the effects of life stresses and disease.

Berk et al. (1989) demonstrated that several minutes of laughter in subjects viewing a humorous film led to lowered epinephrine and cortisol levels, suggesting that immune cells and organs may also have been affected. Although very different from induced laughter, an 8-week course of mindfulness meditation compared to being on a waiting list for meditation training was found to improve immune system response to influenza vaccine (Davidson et al., 2003). Most interestingly, the immune response difference was related to electroencephalographic changes in brain function. These changes are also known to be related to current and tonic positive moods. Another study indicated that the effects of emotional expression could ameliorate the effects of trauma, leading to improved psychological status and immune function. Students were asked to write about either traumatic events in their lives or emotionally neutral events every day for 4 days. Six months later, those who expressed themselves about their traumas were happier and less depressed. They also had better lymphocyte activity, suggesting improved immune function relative to controls (Keller et al., 1994).

Michael Antoni (2003) has explored stress reduction techniques as a means of improving immune system indicators in patients infected with HIV. Patients participating in a 10-week cognitive-behavioral stress management program show improved mood, lower indices of HPAC and sympathetic nervous system activity, lower evidence of viral reactivation, and improved complements of T cells.

Collectively, these studies suggest a potentially beneficial effect on immune system function by use of stress reduction, mood enhancement, and improvements in psychological health. These positive indicators suggest that research on ways to implement interventions to improve health through better immune system functioning may have benefit in specific groups who need such interventions.

Discussion

We began by noting that the immune system is affected by the response to other stressors and that activation of the immune system to fight an infection is in itself a form of stress response. This interplay between immune system and stress-related mechanisms is mirrored by a set of immune-behavioral interactions. On the surface, it is quite remarkable that such interactions should occur at all.

Most psychologists and biologists have held an implicit, strongly dualistic notion of biology and behavior. On the one hand, immunologists have been concerned with hormonal and cellular mechanisms that protect us from invading organisms. These mechanisms have been seen to be highly autonomous, operating without our awareness or conscious control. On the other hand, psychologists have been interested in the conscious and not-so-conscious ways we direct our overt and covert behaviors to operate in the world. The emotions and conscious experiences that accompany and serve these behaviors are a large part of what we call our psychology. And, in a sort of crude computer analogy, psychologists have thought of our bodies as the hardware and our psychology as the software running through, and even controlling, the hardware but not changing the hardware. In other words, neither the behavioral community nor the biological community has been prepared to grasp the full implications of the emerging view that our immune system and our behavior are not separate entities sharing the same space but different expressions of the same biobehavioral process.

If we say that our immune system and our behavior are really only different ways of seeing the same survival process, we begin to recognize that behavior affects our health in a very basic way, by modulating the very system that fights invading organisms. Just as importantly, we recognize that our state of health, and immune function, affects our emotions and behavior. The details of this interplay are becoming increasingly well understood, contributing to a growing reformulation of our dualistic ideas about biology and behavior.

The model of immune response to viral challenge is particularly useful for illustrating the relationship between stress and changes in immune function. The end point of these studies allows clearer interpretations about the changed immune status of the individual as a function of stress. Studies of organ or cell function are less clearly interpretable in terms of global health consequences of immune status.

Also, many lab-based studies use stressors that are at best moderately stressful and emotionally neutral or mildly aversive (e.g., demanding work on a mental arithmetic task). The ability to extrapolate to real-life disasters and severely aversive situations is limited.

At present, we have an increasingly appealing case that emotions and cognitions can alter the function of the immune system. Whether these can alter short-term or long-term health is less certain. The mechanisms by which these connections may come about remain to be explored.

Summary

The immune system is a highly evolved collection of structural defense mechanisms, specialized cells, and chemical messengers. Together, these allow us to survive in a hostile environment containing viruses, bacteria, and other harmful foreign material. The immune system operates in two-way communication with the brain and the endocrine system. Because of this extensive communication, the immune system can influence how we feel and behave. Similarly, our behavior affects the operation of the immune system. Negative emotional states involving feelings of distress are associated with endocrine and autonomic changes that can inhibit immune system function. This results in decreased resistance to new infections and reactivation of latent infections. Studies of humans exposed to brief and prolonged stressors illustrate an array of specific immune alterations and lower resistance to disease. There are also a few encouraging studies suggesting that positive emotional experiences and strong social support networks can enhance immune system function and perhaps improve health.

Further Reading

Ader, R., Felten, D. L., & Cohen, N. (Eds.). *Psychoneuroimmunology* (3rd ed.). New York: Academic Press.

An updated edition of the editors' classic volume on psychoneuroimmunology, an advanced work dealing with a wide range of general themes and specialized topics.

Kiecolt-Glaser, J. K., McGuire, L., Robles, T. F., & Glaser, R. (2002). Psychoneuroimmunology and psychosomatic medicine: Back to the future. *Psychosomatic Medicine, 64,* 15–28.

A review of studies on psychological-immune interactions from 1939 to 2001.

Kuby, J. (1994). *Immunology* (2nd ed.). New York: W. H. Freeman.

A well-illustrated and thorough textbook on immunology.

Glaser, R., & Kiecolt-Glaser, J. K. (Eds.). (1994). *Handbook of human stress and immunity.* San Diego: Academic Press.

A very thorough coverage of topics in stress and immune system function with a heavy emphasis on human work in behavioral medicine.

Rabin, B. (1999). *Stress, immune function and health: The connection.* New York: Wiley-Liss.

A textbook of psychoneuroimmunology with coverage of immune system function and a range of specialized topics on behavior-immune interactions.

Vitaliano, P. P., Zhang, J., & Scanlon, J. (2003). Is caregiving hazardous to one's physical health? A meta-analysis. *Psychological Bulletin, 129,* 946–972.

A thorough review of the literature on the stress of caregiving and its impact on health status.

9

Helplessness, Coping, and Health

In Chapter 6, we presented Lazarus and Folkman's (1984) model of the psychological stress response. That model emphasized perceived control over the environment as a critical determinant of the psychological impact of events. We will now discuss the physiological effects of extreme loss of control in animal and human studies. These form a basis for thinking about the more limited loss of control people often experience as they encounter events in daily life. We will consider two major brainstem systems that may mediate widespread influences of severe stress on emotions, sympathetic outflow, and health. These are the noradrenergic locus ceruleus system and the serotonergic raphe nuclei. Considering the effects of perceived loss of control will add a dimension to our basic question of how ideas can come to have power over the body.

Death Due to Uncontrollable Stress

To emphasize the importance of controllability over events and the ability to master the environment, we begin by considering death—the most extreme result of psychological stress. In an article titled "'Voodoo' Death," Walter Cannon (1957) recounted reports of persons dying because they believed that someone had cast a spell on them and that they had no chance of surviving. In preliterate societies, persons are apt to believe that good and evil forces inhabit the world and that some persons have the ability to harness the evil forces to harm others. Cannon noted reports of the casting of spells and the victims' resulting extreme fear and hopelessness:

> Dr. Lambert . . . wrote to me concerning the experience of Dr. P. S. Clarke. . . . One day a Kanaka came to his hospital and told him he would die in a few days because a spell had been put upon him and nothing could be done to counteract it. The man had been known by Dr. Clarke for some time. He was given a very thorough examination, including an examination of the stool and the urine. All was found normal, but as he lay in bed he gradually grew weaker. Dr. Clarke called upon the foreman of the Kanakas to come to the hospital to give the man assurance, but on reaching the foot of the bed, the foreman leaned over, looked at the patient, and then turned to Dr. Clarke saying, "Yes, doctor, close up him he die." The next day, at 11 o'clock in the morning, he ceased to live. A postmortem examination could reveal nothing that could in any way account for the fatal outcome. (pp. 183–84)

There are common characteristics to Cannon's instances of voodoo death. The victims believed in magic and believed that a specific fatal threat was present and that no escape was possible. This belief system is central to shaping the primary and secondary appraisals laid out in our description of psychological stress in Chapter 6. The very great difference in power between the victim and the forces arrayed against him would have led to the feeling that no effective coping response was available. The psychological origin of this form of death is strongly suggested by the rapid reversal of the process when the occasional victim was convinced that the evil spell had been lifted. Cannon speculated that the profound feelings of hopelessness engendered in the victims of voodoo death resulted in severe metabolic and autonomic imbalances, often accompanied by failure to take in nutrients, resulting in death within days to weeks. These examples are strong testimony to the considerable influence of our beliefs in shaping neurophysiological patterns and the descending bodily outputs that accompany them.

Sudden Death Due to Uncontrollable Stress

The examples of voodoo death may sound exotic and irrelevant to modern life. Nevertheless, there are numerous recent examples of sudden death precipitated by psychological causes. Engel (1971) did an extensive search of newspaper accounts of persons dying suddenly under extreme circumstances. In most cases, the victim had experienced a personal loss, such as death of a spouse or child or separation from a loved one. Often the person had a restricted range of social contacts and experienced the loss as irreplaceable and severe. Still other persons were faced with an exceptionally difficult personal dilemma in which the available courses of action all led to undesirable outcomes. In other cases, a violently emotional confrontation, often involving the severing of strong personal ties, preceded the sudden death, or the person had returned home to discover that his or her house had been burglarized and ransacked.

Certainly, the emotional content differed in the various incidents Engel reported. Nevertheless, the emotions were all *powerful negative* ones, including anger and fear, and death appeared to be preceded by overwhelming feelings of *helplessness* or *hopelessness*. In cases where medical information was available, the cause of death was most often attributable to massive myocardial infarction or cerebrovascular stroke. Although Engel's examples tend to be anecdotal, their lifelike character lends them credibility.

Recent patient reports show that the likelihood of a heart attack is about two times greater than usual in the 2 hours following an episode of anger (Mittleman et al., 1995). Reports of sudden coronary death and stroke can rise substantially during times of increased threat to the population. During the Los Angeles earthquake of 1994, more than half of all immediate deaths were due to sudden cardiac death, not to injuries. Death records showed that sudden coronary deaths were five times greater than expected on the day of the earthquake (Leor, Poole, & Kloner, 1996). During Operation Desert Storm in 1991, deaths rose dramatically in Israel during the Iraqi Scud missile attacks. In targeted cities, death rates due to heart attack and related causes were more than twice normal (Kark, Goldman, & Epstein, 1995). Not all cardiac episodes result from genuine disasters; some result from events interpreted as such by the victims. Carroll, Ebrahim, Tilling, Macleod, and Smith (2002) found that English hospital admissions for myocardial infarction rose above normal for 3 days in 1998 following Britain's unexpected loss to Argentina in a World Cup soccer match. These examples indicate that severely threatening circumstances having a rapid onset can lead to apparent or documented coronary events and stroke.

Other uncontrollable stressors may act more slowly and through different mechanisms to affect health. Being exposed daily to a crowded environment with attendant opportunities for irritating and hostile encounters may also form a health hazard. Cristenfeld and colleagues found that residents of New York die at 155% of the expected rate, visitors die while in the city at 134% of the expected rate, but New Yorkers visiting elsewhere die at only 80% of the expected rate. New York City was rated the fifth most stressful major city in a recent survey of stressful social and environmental urban characteristics (Christenfeld, Glynn, Phillips, & Shrira, 1999). To take a very different example, investigators in Denmark carried out a long-term follow-up of parents who had experienced the death of a child and found that bereaved mothers had 3.8 times the expected rate of death from unnatural causes in the first 3 years following their loss (Li, Precht, Mortensen, & Olsen, 2003). During the 10th to 18th years of follow-up, these women still experienced a 44% increase in deaths due to natural causes.

This evidence suggests that psychological stress can be associated with increased morbidity and mortality. The precipitating event may be a natural disaster, extreme fear introduced by uncontrollable threat, or grief at the loss of a child. The common theme is that all these events threaten well-being through psychological means and have a degree of uncontrollability. They are seen to violate the affected individual's life expectations, goals, and commitments, and they appear to leave the individual limited opportunities for coping.

Possible Mechanisms of Sudden Death

Figure 9.1 illustrates five major steps by which overwhelming uncontrollable threat can lead to sudden death:

1. Contact with an uncontrollable aversive event triggers primary threat appraisals, secondary appraisals that coping resources are limited, and negative emotions, as described in Figure 6.1.

2. Such emotions can significantly increase autonomic outflow to the peripheral organs and secretion of the stress-related hormones epinephrine and cortisol.

3. These autonomic and endocrine changes can increase the demand of the heart muscle for oxygen, increase stress on the walls of the blood vessels due to elevated blood pressure, and enhance the formation of blood clots.

4. Vascular stress, along with increased clotting, increases the risk of cerebrovascular stroke. Cardiac stress increases the risk of myocardial infarction and left ventricular arrhythmias leading to ventricular fibrillation.

5. Stroke, myocardial infarction, and ventricular arrhythmia are the most common causes of sudden death.

Arrows do not connect the boxes in Figure 9.1 because the specific relationships among them are multiple.

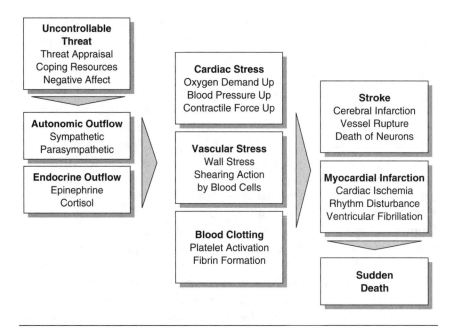

Figure 9.1   Events leading from uncontrollable psychological stress to sudden death.

Stress-induced fatal heart attacks or strokes occur most often in persons who already have atherosclerosis of the coronary arteries or arteriosclerosis of the arteries supplying the brain. The buildup of arterial plaque has several consequences:

1. The plaque narrows the vessel, resulting in episodes of ischemia (a lack of sufficient oxygen delivery to the tissues) when stress leads to increased oxygen demand.

2. The affected blood vessels are especially subject to the formation of blood clots, blocking the vessel and causing ischemia and possible myocardial infarction or stroke.

3. The plaque weakens the blood vessel wall, with the risk of arterial rupture, again leading to infarction or stroke. All these consequences of stress can result in ischemia and possible tissue damage.

Stress-induced arrhythmia of the heart can also result from ischemia and result in sudden cardiac death. Cardiac muscle ischemia during increased oxygen demand can lead to a loss of normal cardiac rhythm, resulting in ventricular tachycardia (rapid, but coordinated, contraction of the left ventricle out of synchrony with the rest of the heart), followed by left ventricular fibrillation (uncoordinated ventricular contractions). This causes the heart to fail to pump effectively, leading to loss of consciousness and death.

The etiology of sudden cardiac death due to emotional influences has been studied extensively in animal models by Bernard Lown, Richard Verrier, and colleagues (Saini & Verrier, 1989) and has been reviewed from a psychosocial perspective by Kamarck and Jennings (1991). Lampert et al. (2002) have studied the relationship between mental stress and aggravation of underlying arrhythmias in persons with cardiac disease. Their work showed that mental stress can increase the risk for ventricular tachycardia and sudden death in the absence of physical exertion. Blumenthal et al. (1995) have pointed out that episodes of myocardial ischemia in daily life are usually not associated with physical exertion and are presumably associated with other factors, such as emotional distress, that may elicit symptoms. Patients with known heart disease who have myocardial ischemia during mental stress evaluation in the laboratory are more likely to have ischemic episodes and coronary events in their daily lives (Jiang et al., 1996). The secretion of epinephrine, an important concomitant of emotional distress, such as fear and anger, can potentiate all the lethal outcomes that ensue during acute emotional distress. Circulating epinephrine can lead to clot formation, increased blood pressure resulting in stroke, or extreme increases in the demand of the heart muscle for oxygen, even at rest (Sung, Wilson, Robinson, Thadani, & Lovallo, 1988). Krantz, Quigley, and O'Callahan (2001) have recently reviewed the use of laboratory-based mental stress challenges to study these relationships.

We strongly suspect that in many, if not most, cases of human sudden death, the person has unrecognized, preexisting coronary artery disease or an arrhythmia-prone heart muscle. In such persons, large increases in myocardial oxygen demand would lead to ischemia of the heart muscle, increasing the risk of myocardial infarction, lethal arrhythmia, or both. Sudden, overwhelming emotions, especially uncontrolled fear and anger, could act to produce a myocardial infarction or an episode of ischemia or could trigger a lethal arrhythmia in a person with preexisting disease. In a study of 19 cases of sudden, unexplained death, five cases had known prior symptoms, such as fainting, or documented cardiac functional disturbances, such as tachycardia, indicating underlying cardiac pathology. In four deaths where there was a clear precipitating factor, two were preceded by exercise and the other two were preceded by episodes of emotional distress (Morentin, Suarez-Mier, & Aguilera, 2003). Risk factors for sudden cardiac arrest among persons with known coronary artery disease are prior myocardial infarction, hypertension, and heavy coffee consumption (de Vreede-Swagemakers et al., 1999). Nonetheless, the presence of prior disease or poor dietary habits in cases of sudden death should not divert our attention from the role of the individual's perception of the environment, interpretation of events, and emotional response as immediately precipitating factors. Evidence is emerging that clinical events can be reduced over a period of years by training heart disease patients to cognitively regulate their emotional responses during potentially stressful episodes (Blumenthal et al., 2002).

Helplessness and Exposure to Uncontrollable Stress

Most episodes of loss of control do not result in death. Nevertheless, we suspect that a sense of reduced control in the face of perceived threat occurs commonly in the daily lives of many of us, and it is desirable to know its effects. Laboratory work on these topics has had an interesting history, and selected examples suggest that this work has led to a better understanding of the effects of uncontrollable stress on behavior, emotions, brain chemistry, and immune function.

To study uncontrollable stress and its effect on health, Joseph Brady and colleagues tested yoked-control pairs of rhesus monkeys using a procedure known as a Sidman avoidance paradigm (Brady, Porter, Conrad, & Mason, 1958). This task calls for a subject to make avoidance responses, such as pressing a bar, every so often or else to receive some aversive consequence, usually a shock, if the response is not made on schedule. This is highly stressful in the long run because the subject must be vigilant to respond appropriately. There are inevitable lapses of attention that result in shock delivery, but these will occur unpredictably from the subject's point of view. The use of a yoked control indicates that one animal is chosen to make the avoidance responses while the other receives all the same shocks and can press a bar, but this does not actually control the shock presentation. In Brady's study, pairs of animals received a low-level electric shock every 20 seconds unless the "Executive" monkey pressed a bar and postponed the shock for 20 more seconds. The yoked monkey also had a bar but could not influence the shocks. This procedure continued for 6 hours on and 6 hours off without interruption. The Executive monkeys all died with gastric ulcers after 9 to 48 days on this unremitting schedule.

This study attracted a great deal of attention. Ulcers were a serious disorder in the 1950s, prior to the advent of effective medications. The popular stereotype of the day was that harried executives were the ones most likely to develop ulcers as a result of the stressful, dominant role they held, having to make important decisions and be responsible for their subordinates. So the study of these Executive monkeys and their yoked pair-mates seemed to have a special relevance to everyday life.

However, recall that the yoked and Executive monkeys received the same shocks. According to our model of psychological stress, the yoked (helpless) monkeys should experience greater loss of control and should therefore be under greater stress. Why did these monkeys not show ulceration and death? It turns out that there was a flaw in the execution of the study—the most active monkeys were systematically assigned to the Executive role. To facilitate the experiment, Brady had cut one critical corner, failing to randomly assign animals to their roles in the yoked pairs. Instead, he pretested all the monkeys in the avoidance apparatus to find those that would press the bar spontaneously and at a steady rate, and then he assigned these to the role of Executive monkey. The Executive monkeys were therefore spontaneously active, and perhaps reactive, having a spontaneous bar press rate of 15 to 20 responses per minute, whereas the yoked monkeys were by default less active and more placid in the face of the shocks. In following up on these initial findings, neither Brady nor others could replicate the results.

What made this research interesting, even though the results were misleading, was that it illustrated how psychological stress could be manipulated to differ between the two animals while the physical stress of the electric shock could be held constant. This paradigm would later show the importance of psychological variables in determining the consequences of exposure to a shock stressor, and it produced valuable information on the central nervous system mechanisms that were involved. We will review these studies selectively and briefly.

We should note in passing that the ulcers caused in animals by uncontrollable shock are not the same kind that human ulcer sufferers have. The ulcers seen in stressed animals are interesting to stress researchers because they are manifestations of Selye's general adaptation syndrome. Gastric ulcers are known to be inducible by electrical stimulation of the amygdala, but they do not tell us about the true possible somatic or psychosomatic causes of human ulcers (Weiner, 1991a, 1991b). We now know that most human ulcers are caused by reactivation of a chronic gastric infection by the bacterium *Helicobacter pylori*. Although it is possible that bacterial reactivation is related to episodes of stress, this link has yet to be established. Susan Levenstein (2000) provides a current account of the relationship between emotional distress and activity of gastric ulcers in the human population.

Studies of Ulceration in Rats

In pursuing the interesting leads from Brady et al.'s monkey experiments, Jay Weiss and colleagues tested the effects of exposure to uncontrollable shock in rats. These studies are relevant to the effects of stress in humans because they suggest that the *meaning* of external events can alter their impact on the individual. In so doing, they tell us how psychological influences can modulate the physical consequences of stress.

Predictability as a Moderator of Physical Consequences of Stress

In understanding the stress-buffering effects of coping processes, it is useful to know if predicting the timing of an aversive event reduces its negative effects even if it cannot be avoided. Accordingly, Weiss (1970) examined whether warning animals of impending electric shocks could reduce their physiological effects. In his first study, predictability was manipulated in three groups of animals. One group was handled and placed in the experimental apparatus but never actually shocked, another received randomly scheduled shocks to the tail, and the third group received the same tail shocks, but each shock was preceded by a 10-second warning tone. The percentage of rats in each group that developed stress-induced ulcers differed markedly: 25% among the no-shock controls, 67% in those given a warning tone, and 100% of the unpredictably shocked rats. The unpredictably shocked animals also had the highest body temperatures, lost the most weight, and secreted the most corticosterone (the rat equivalent of cortisol). This suggests that the amygdala and central corticotropin releasing factor system, as discussed in Chapters 6 and 7, were differentially activated in the animals deprived of the ability to predict shocks.

Because the amount of shock was identical between the two shock groups, the increased corticosterone secretion was considered to result from differences in perception of the stressful situation in the unsignaled animals. Even though the rats could not control the shocks, it was clear that the physical consequences of this stressor could be buffered by forewarning that the shock was about to occur.

Weiss concluded that the warning signal also provided a safety signal by its very absence, allowing the intervals before the tones to become safe periods. In a second study, Weiss found that the safety of these periods could be contaminated. In this case, he filled the interval between tones with a long-lasting, gradually increasing tone that culminated in a shock.

In fact, the warning tone became a conditioned stimulus, signaling impending danger throughout most of the interval between shocks and leading to high rates of ulceration. Clearly, the tone became a signal for danger, not a sign of safety. Both studies had a common theme: The psychological nuances of the situation were a major determinant of the physical outcome of the stressful events.

Controllability as a Moderator of Physical Effects of Stress

Given these striking effects of predictability, Weiss (1971a) next examined the ulcer-buffering effects of control over aversive events. He used a *triadic design* based on a traditional yoked-control model. Groups of three animals were placed in individual plastic test chambers with their tails and tail-shock electrodes extending out a hole in the back. One animal, whose electrode was not connected to the shock apparatus, served as an unshocked control for the effects of handling and apparatus exposure. The other two were yoked to receive identical electric shocks. One of these, designated the Executive rat, could avoid shocks by turning a wheel; the other was the helpless, yoked control. They underwent a Sidman avoidance paradigm in which the Executive rat could avoid shocks for itself and its yoked partner by turning a wheel with its forepaws. The Executive rats got far fewer ulcers than the helpless rats, apparently because they could control shocks. The yoked rats were helpless to avoid shock, and their wheel turning was unrelated to the presentation of absence of shock. The results are shown in the left set of bars in Figure 9.2 (the No Signal condition). Weiss (1971b) also showed that providing appropriate warning signals could further reduce the impact of the shocks on ulcer formation (the Signal condition, Figure 9.2). Therefore, both control and predictability were capable of acting as stress buffers, modulating the impact of the aversive events.

These results are opposite to the ones Brady reported in his monkeys. Instead of the overworked Executives having ulcers, it was the helpless animals, unable to cope with the shocks, that felt the greatest impact. This finding fits with the model of psychological stress described in Chapter 6. Events should have a greater negative impact on an animal when no coping behavior is available. So we can see that the control afforded the Executive rat buffers the effect of the stressor by providing a means of coping.

With regard to Brady's earlier work, when Weiss reanalyzed the data for all the animals in his study, the ones that had the highest spontaneous rates of wheel turning also had the most ulcers, regardless of which condition

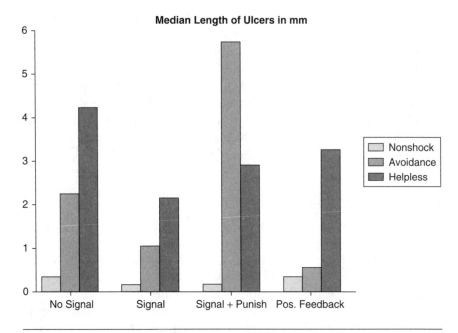

Median Length of Ulcers in mm

Legend:
- Nonshock
- Avoidance
- Helpless

X-axis: No Signal   Signal   Signal + Punish   Pos. Feedback

Figure 9.2   Ulcers in relation to control and quality of feedback in rats. Redrawn from Weiss (1971a, 1971b).

they were in. This lends credence to the criticism of Brady's nonrandom assignment of high-responding monkeys to the Executive monkey role.

Positive Feedback as a Moderator of Stress Responses

In related studies, Weiss investigated the effects of positive and negative consequences of a successful avoidance response on the amount of ulceration in the Executive animals (Weiss, 1971b). In one condition, the Executive and control rats were given a very brief shock each time they performed an avoidance response. This punishment in conjunction with a correct avoidance response resulted in the Executive rats having more ulcers than the helpless rats, even though they were in fact in control and avoiding the longer shocks that would otherwise have occurred (the Signal + Punish condition, Figure 9.2). On the other hand, when the rats were given a tone signaling that the Executive rat had successfully avoided the next shock by turning the wheel, their ulcers were almost totally eliminated (the Pos. Feedback condition, Figure 9.2).

The general conclusion from this work is that the psychological concomitants of the situation can enhance or reduce the effects of the stressor on the individual. We might say that the primary cause of the negative physical consequences of the shock in these studies is not the shock itself. Instead, the physical outcomes depend greatly on the psychological impact of the event. Further, although these studies tell us why and how stressors can be bad for us, they also tell us how psychological buffers, such as information about safety and successful avoidance, can modulate the impact of negative events.

Learned Helplessness and the Consequences of Lack of Control

About the time Weiss was carrying out these studies in his rats, Martin Seligman, Stephen Maier, and Richard Solomon (1971) were exploring other aspects of uncontrollable stress in a series of studies on dogs. In this work, dogs were suspended individually in hammocks to hold them in position during administration of inescapable shocks. There were three groups: a hammock-only control group, an avoidance group that could avoid the presentation of periodic shocks by pressing a plate with their noses, and a helpless yoked-control group. The animals were retested 24 hours later in a shuttle box avoidance procedure.

The shuttle box consisted of two chambers separated by a low barrier. Shocks were provided to the dogs' feet by a metal grid that formed the floor of the chambers, and the shocks were signaled by a brief tone. In this training, dogs learn within a few trials to leap over the barrier to the safety of the other chamber. In fact, the control and avoidance groups from the prior training did just that. However, the animals that were unable to control the shocks in the sling training were almost completely unable to learn this simple avoidance behavior.

Seligman and his coworkers observed marked emotional changes in the helpless dogs: They exhibited greater fearfulness and anxiety. When placed in the shuttle training apparatus, they cowered in one side of the box and allowed themselves to be shocked rather than learning to jump the barrier. Seligman used the term *learned helplessness* to characterize the cognitive, emotional, and performance deficits shown by the dogs after exposure to uncontrollable shock. They theorized that this apparent helplessness develops when outcomes (shocks) are not contingent on performance (attempts at escape or avoidance). The instrumental independence of an avoidance attempt and its outcome was presumed to result in the shocked animal learning a specific lack of dependence of outcomes on behavior, resulting in a lasting, learned deficit in the dog's ability to learn new avoidance behaviors. This learning-based formulation was bolstered by the observation that dogs bred and reared in a kennel were more susceptible to uncontrollable shock effects than captured mongrel dogs. The mongrels presumably were *immunized* by their history of successful coping with the environment outside the laboratory.

Seligman and colleagues argued that exposure to uncontrollable shock has four major consequences: (a) The animal develops an expectation that its responses are independent of the outcomes; (b) response initiation is reduced because responses have failed to produce consistent outcomes in the past; (c) such animals are less able to learn to respond correctly in similar situations; and (d) depression may ensue. In short, it appeared that the animals had learned to be helpless and that this experience led to depression. Seligman et al. (1971) therefore termed this the *learned helplessness model of depression.*

Although this learning-based model of the behavioral effects of uncontrollable shock exposure was appealing, there were other viable formulations. First, Weiss noted that the dissipation of the effect over time (approximately 48–72 hours) by his rats, and Seligman's dogs, argued against a learned deficit, which should have been more permanent. Second, the deficit in Weiss's rats was associated with a reduction of central nervous system norepinephrine (NE). These discrepancies led Weiss to propose a *motor activation deficit* model of uncontrollable stress. Under this model, uncontrollable stress was said to result in depletion of central nervous system NE, leading to decreased response initiation and hence motor activation deficits.

Weiss (1980) first conducted a series of studies to contrast the effects of uncontrollability per se from the effects of stress. To do so, he exposed rats to a helplessness-inducing swim test in a glass cylinder half filled with water and having smooth walls. The stressfulness of the experience could be manipulated independently by altering the water temperature. This model therefore allowed the effect of stress to be evaluated independently of uncontrollability. Rats exposed to the swim test in the less stressful room-temperature water had no deficit later in a rat analogue of the shuttle box task used in dogs. In contrast, rats exposed to a highly stressful cold-water swim showed the expected deficit. Clearly, in the face of equal uncontrollability, the behavioral deficit only occurred when stress levels were high.

The cold swim also increased the performance-retarding effect of placing a higher barrier in the shuttle box, but it did not prevent learning to climb the barrier to avoid, again favoring the performance deficit hypothesis. Similarly, the cold swim did not interfere with learning behaviors that were very easy to perform, such as a nose poke to avoid shock. Inescapable shock functioned the same as the cold swim; it reduced shuttle box performance but did not produce a nose-poke deficit. Fourteen sessions of cold swim abolished the shuttling deficit, a result incompatible with the rats learning to be helpless. The same stress immunization occurred with 14 sessions of inescapable shock, again arguing against a learned form of helplessness.

These studies convincingly argued that the deficit in establishing avoidance behaviors after inescapable shock was due to a performance deficit associated with the level of the stress. With shock held constant, greater levels of stress were experienced by the helpless animals. With helplessness held constant, the performance deficit was worse with increasing stress.

Other evidence showed that the effects of the cold swim dissipated over 48 hours, enough time for the locus ceruleus to synthesize more NE. Studies by Weiss later showed that the performance deficit increased as central NE declined and decreased as the NE recovered. Shuttle box deficits following either uncontrollable shock or cold swim were not due to changes in other central transmitters, such as serotonin, dopamine, or acetylcholine (Weiss et al., 1981). Weiss was able to mimic the effects of inescapable shock or cold swim by directly manipulating locus ceruleus NE. Chemical depletion of NE led to shuttle box deficits. Repeated depletion of NE did not produce shuttle box deficits. Monoamine oxidase inhibitors, drugs that reduce the breakdown of NE, counteracted the shuttle box deficit following inescapable shock.

Central Neurotransmitters and Severe Stress

How would central NE become depleted by stress, and why would such a depletion alter motor activation? As noted in Chapter 6, the primary source of central NE is the noradrenergic cell bodies of the locus ceruleus of the pons. This critical nucleus communicates with the entire central nervous system. It produces a steady firing rate, thought to act as a central pacemaker, setting the background level of CNS activity. When alerted by signals from the amygdala (see Figure 6.3), the locus ceruleus increases its firing rate, resulting in increased alerting of the forebrain and limbic system. During transient threats, this is an adaptive means of alerting the central nervous system. However, longer-term disruption of locus ceruleus firing patterns by NE depletion would chronically alter the timing of ascending activation. This would alter the ability of the prefrontal cortex, amygdala, and hippocampus to evaluate incoming stimuli and would disrupt the formulation and initiation of behavioral responses until the activation pattern returned to normal.

The locus ceruleus contains two sets of NE-synthesizing neurons. One set projects outward to all parts of the central nervous system (see Figure 6.4). The other set consists of small, inhibitory interneurons that internally modulate the firing of the other set. During uncontrollable shock exposure, the locus ceruleus receives high levels of input from the amygdala and hypothalamus, resulting in high firing rates. Eventually, this high level of activity depletes NE stores selectively in the smaller inhibitory interneurons. This loss of internal inhibition results in the ascending neurons producing frequent, abnormally long bursts of activity. Because of the locus ceruleus's ability to modulate sensory processes and prefrontal-limbic communication, it is plausible that stress-induced activation of the locus ceruleus would have significant emotional and behavioral consequences. Extensive coverage of studies manipulating locus ceruleus NE is provided in several reviews (Weiss, 1991; Weiss et al., 1981).

Uncontrollable Shock, Norepinephrine, and Depression

Related work by Weiss showed that both exposure to uncontrollable shock and chemical manipulation of NE in the locus ceruleus led to behavioral changes corresponding to six of the eight clinical signs of human depression. These were (a) poor appetite and weight loss; (b) poor performance on tasks requiring psychomotor performance; (c) loss of energy and apparent fatigue; (d) loss of interest in usual activities (in rats this means grooming, aggressiveness, and competitiveness); (e) sleep changes, including less sleep time and more fragmented sleep; and (f) increased distractibility and indecision (Weiss, Simson, Ambrose, Webster, & Hoffman, 1985). As we know, the other two symptoms of human depression, thoughts of suicide and feelings of worthlessness, are not observable in rats.

One can view these studies as favoring the development of depression due to central nervous system alterations associated with uncontrollable stress. However, this work leaves major questions about the etiology of depression unanswered. Weiss's animals did not show alterations in the serotonin-containing raphe nuclei, although there is evidence that these are important in mood disturbances (Williams, 1994). Also, the dissipation of the behavioral deficit in dogs and rats after 48 to 72 hours differs from the relatively long-lasting mood and behavioral changes associated with clinical depression in humans.

With such limitations in mind, these studies are significant because they show that the brainstem nuclei are responsive to psychological characteristics of the stressful situation. The outcome of this organism-environment interaction is a major determinant of subsequent behavior and moods. Most important for our present concern with psychological stress, it appears that the impact of an uncontrollable stressor on the individual depends heavily on the interpretation given to the situation and the coping options available. The effects of intermittent uncontrollable shock depend on the animal's being conscious, further supporting the interpretation that these effects are due to the psychological aspects of the situation.

In Chapter 6, we outlined central mechanisms of the stress response. We noted the relationship between interpretations of the world and the activity of important emotion-controlling centers of the temporal lobes. These data suggest that manipulating the interpretation of the events experienced in the course of exposure to aversive events can have powerful affective and behavioral consequences.

Serotonin Mechanisms

Although Weiss's work on behavioral depression and uncontrollable aversive stress favored the view that the locus ceruleus was the critical site of altered central nervous system function, other work suggests that social stress can alter the serotonergic system associated with the brainstem raphe nuclei. Like the locus ceruleus, the raphe nuclei send fibers to many sites in the central nervous system. Descending fibers activate the motor neurons of the spinal cord, and ascending fibers travel to all parts of the cortex and to the hippocampus and amygdala. Drugs that alter serotonin levels in the brain affect moods and behaviors, including feelings of depression but also hostility, anger, and aggression. In recent years, treatments for mood disorders have included drugs that enhance the availability of serotonin at the synapse. Of interest to us, there is evidence that stress may alter serotonin levels.

Uncontrollable social stress, especially early in life, may produce long-standing reductions in serotonin with consequent changes in behavior and emotions. In one group of studies, rhesus monkeys were separated from their mothers very early in life and placed in social groups consisting entirely of similarly displaced young. These social groups are highly disrupted and do not have the normal status hierarchy that results from having members of different ages. As a result, there is a great deal of unresolved conflict and social disorganization. In studies by Linnoila and colleagues, young monkeys were placed in peer-only groups and lived there continuously prior to their introduction into normal, hierarchical social groups at 6 months of age. These peer-reared monkeys had decreased serotonin levels that persisted at least until 5 years of age. They had defective social interactions, including excessive aggression and less affiliation with others. These maternally deprived monkeys also showed exaggerated cortisol responses during social interactions (Higley, Suomi, & Linnoila, 1992). This work suggests that the stress of loss of nurturance and exposure to high levels of social disruption has a long-lasting effect on brain serotonin and behavior. Both the locus ceruleus and serotonergic nuclei appear to respond to uncontrollable stress exposure by reduced availability of their respective neurotransmitters. These changes pervasively modulate behavior, emotion, and stress proneness.

Emotions and Health

The above animal work suggests potent, possibly chronic effects of uncontrollable stress on the central mechanisms of behavior, mood, and neuroendocrine function. In addition, intermittent, uncontrollable shock suppresses immune function (Weiss & Sundar, 1992). Therefore, we may ask whether feelings of helplessness or hopelessness are related to health in a more direct way. Although evidence in humans has been difficult to obtain, recent work suggests that negative moods, a common outcome of reduced control over life events, may be associated with poorer health outcomes.

Depression and hostility were significantly related to a variety of negative health outcomes in an extensive reanalysis of data from a large number of studies (Booth-Kewley & Friedman, 1987). In a longitudinal study, hostility predicted increased risk of coronary artery disease and mortality due to all causes (Barefoot, Dahlstrom, & Williams, 1983). Hostility during midlife, and increases in hostility over time, predict poorer health indicators, such as low social support, social isolation, low income, and obesity (Siegler et al., 2003). Depressed elderly persons may have a suppression of their immune systems, leaving them exposed to increased risk of infection and cancer (Solomon & Benton, 1994). As noted in Chapter 8, elderly caregivers had reduced immune system function, indexed by slow wound healing, and younger subjects who reported higher levels of life stress, low social support, and more negative affect also evidenced impaired immune system function.

Recent epidemiologic work suggests that feelings of hopelessness are related to increased risk of death due to various causes. Everson and colleagues studied a cohort of 2,428 men from eastern Finland and followed their health status for 6 years. At the beginning of the study these men answered the questions "I feel that it is impossible to reach the goals I should like to strive for" and "The future seems to me to be hopeless, and I can't believe that things are changing for the better," using scales of agreement ranging from 0 to 4. The cohort was divided into men scoring low (0–2), medium (3–5), and high (6–8) on the two items combined. Hopelessness scores were related in a dose-response fashion to risk of death due to all causes, including violent death and injury, and to incidence of myocardial infarction and cancer (Everson, Goldberg, et al., 1996). Related work from this same cohort showed that among men who had atherosclerosis at the start of the study, those higher in hopelessness had greater worsening of their disease over the 4 years than their more optimistic counterparts (Everson, Kaplan, Goldberg, Salonen, & Salonen, 1997). The more hopeless men also had three times the risk of developing hypertension over a 4-year follow-up (Everson, Kaplan, Goldberg, & Salonen, 2000).

Discussion

The material reviewed in this chapter illustrates major elements of psychological stress processes as outlined in Chapter 6. The central feature of that model is the individual's appraisals of an event and the resources available to control it. These are critical in determining how stressful the event is. Work on aversive stress in animals shows that the psychological elements of the organism-environment interaction, such as novelty and uncontrollability, appear to greatly enhance the stress value of the stimuli and determine their physical consequences. This leads us to the consideration that many of the stressors encountered in modern life, though they pose little physical threat, may have a significant impact on mood and health based on the person's feelings of control.

Feelings of helplessness can greatly alter the effects of aversive events on behavior, mood, and central noradrenergic and serotonergic systems. It is significant that drugs known to alter mood in humans can also alter the physical effects of the stressors in animals. The effects of these drugs parallel their effects on NE and serotonin in the brain, suggesting that the aminergic nuclei are important in the generation of emotions, along with the frontal areas and amygdala. The negative emotion states are of particular concern to our study of the effects of stress on health. They accompany behaviors that put persons at greater risk of violent death. They also predict short-term decreases in immune function and long-term negative health outcomes.

The use of yoked-control designs in animal studies shows clearly that the impact of a physical stressor, such as shock, can be enhanced by lack of controllability but can also be buffered by behavioral control, warning of impending shock, signals indicating success in avoidance, and prior experience. Thus, this work conveys both a negative and a positive message about the effects of stress on health and how they can be lessened.

We have noted in this chapter that the effect of uncontrollable stress in animals may resemble the severe uncontrollability and overpowering emotions experienced by human victims of natural disasters. This work may, in turn, be relevant to an understanding of posttraumatic stress disorder (PTSD). The most important effects of traumatic stress on humans are not its peripheral autonomic and endocrine effects but its effects on the central nervous system. Victims of PTSD manifest exaggerated emotional responses to a wide range of stimuli and show accompanying autonomic changes. The most pervasive and disturbing aspects of the disorder are the occurrence of intrusive thoughts and dysphoric moods, including depression as well as anxiety, persisting for many years after the precipitating events. These changes would appear to be related to enhanced reactivity of amygdala circuits and involving long-term alterations in frontal-limbic connections and alterations in feedback to the central nervous system from the brainstem aminergic nuclei. So we may consider that the central nervous system mechanisms integrating the psychological stress response may undergo long-term changes due to the severe uncontrollability accompanying traumatic stress. These central changes may appear to mediate the most troubling and persistent effects of uncontrollable stress. They may well reflect an alteration of the response bias of the system as a result of extreme levels of stress-related activation.

Turning to the basic question of this book, we asked how ideas can be translated into changes in the body. We have presented increasingly strong evidence that our ability to interpret our world and to invest that interpretation with personal meaning and emotion has a direct and powerful effect on the body. The examples of death due to devastating emotional distress provide testimony to the power of ideas to change our physical well-being. The mechanisms of this translation are being increasingly well established in animal models, and these are finding confirmation in observations of humans in the laboratory and in their daily lives. The sometimes dramatic effects of a traumatic event lead us to recognize that not all persons respond alike. Different persons will interpret the same event in very different ways, with equally different consequences for their well-being. In Chapter 11, we will consider some of the ways that persons differ in their responses to stressful events.

Summary

Psychological stress can lead to severe physical consequences, including death. The model of psychological stress in Chapter 6 suggests that the degree of coping and control available to an individual determines the stressfulness of an event and the physical reactions to it. In contrast, the physical effect of an aversive stressor can be entirely overcome by providing appropriate means of behavioral control and positive feedback for successful coping. Psychological stress is accompanied by negative emotions and associated behaviors including depression, hostility, anger, and aggression. These emotions are heavily influenced by the activity of brainstem adrenergic nuclei that have extensive connections to the frontal areas of the cortex and limbic structures, including the hippocampus and amygdala. These negative emotions appear to be related to immune system function and health outcomes.

Further Reading

Cannon, W. B. (1957). "Voodoo" death. *Psychosomatic Medicine, 19*, 182–190.

An engaging work on the effect of belief systems on physical well-being. Highly recommended as a classic in the stress field.

Weiss, J. M. (1980). Part V: Explaining behavioral depression following uncontrollable stressful events. *Behavioral Research and Therapy, 18*, 485–504.

A highly readable account of Weiss's early work demonstrating an important technique for studying the psychological impact of stress in animals and the role of uncontrollable stress in altering brain chemistry.

Weiss, J. M. (1991). Stress-induced depression: Critical neurochemical and electrophysiological changes (pp. 123–154). In I. J. Madden (Ed.), *Neurobiology of learning, emotion and affect*. New York: Raven.

A detailed account of the alterations in locus ceruleus norepinephrine in behavioral depression and how this results in differential activation of higher centers receiving inputs from the locus ceruleus.

Booth-Kewley, S., & Friedman, H. (1987). Psychological predictors of heart disease: A quantitative review. *Psychological Bulletin, 101,* 343–362.

A major analysis of the relationship between negative emotions and health summarizes a great deal of literature on the subject.

Siegman, A. W., & Smith, T. W. (Eds.). (1994). *Anger, hostility, and the heart.* Hillsdale, NJ: Lawrence Erlbaum.

An extensive coverage of the relationship between hostility and the risk of coronary artery disease.

Saini, V., & Verrier, R. L. (1989). The experimental study of behaviorally induced arrhythmias. In N. Schneiderman, P. Kaufmann, & S. Weiss (Eds.), *Handbook of research methods in cardiovascular behavioral medicine* (pp. 51–68). New York: Plenum.

A very thorough summary of studies on sudden cardiac death due to stress in animal models.

Van Heeringen, K. (2003). The neurobiology of suicide and suicidality. *Canadian Journal of Psychiatry, 48,* 292–300.

A good brief review of the relationship between altered serotonin function and central nervous system activity associated with suicide and underlying behavioral dispositions.

10

Genes, Stress, and Behavior

A persistent question in stress research is how and why persons differ so dramatically in response to potentially threatening events in daily life. What makes one person react with extreme anxiety where another person might merely behave with due caution? Why will one person view an irritable colleague as merely a "character" where another might see this person as an enemy? Perhaps most interestingly, these differences in behavioral tendencies often persist throughout a person's lifetime, and underlying these traits appear to be biologically based differences in temperament. The idea that temperament represents an inborn disposition having a traitlike consistency is reminiscent of the ways that breeds of dogs have relatively stable behavioral tendencies; Labrador retrievers are consistently faithful and solicitous to their owners, Afghan hounds are independent minded, and standard poodles are intelligent but become playful goof-offs when bored during their training exercises. Nevertheless, individual experience is still important; despite their temperamental differences, all of these dogs are better companions and easier to live with when given lots of attention and gentle but firm training as youngsters.

Recent studies of early life experience in animals and humans have begun to yield some insights into how social influences can interact with brain development in ways that direct and redirect emotional responsivity and behavior throughout life. Perhaps most importantly, these same studies are beginning to yield information on environmental influences on gene expression. These developments are therefore important, not only for what they can tell us about emotional disposition and stress reactivity, but because they are the beginning of an era in developmental research that allows us to see the interactions of genes and environment, of nature and nurture. With regard to our present topic of stress and health, they can tell us much about the origins and bases of stress reactivity differences among people. In this chapter, we will spend some time describing the key studies of genes, environment, and the shaping of reactivity to the environment. In Chapter 11, we will lay out a physiologically based model of individual differences in stress reactivity.

Early Life Experience, Gene Expression, and Stress Reactivity

Crime and Punishment: Rooster Bogle and the Bogle Clan

Dale Vincent Bogle, known as "Rooster," was born in Texas in 1941. He had a history of arrests as a young man, including domestic violence and stealing, and served time in prison before he was 19. After moving to Oregon, he continued his lifestyle while encouraging his children to do the same. The *New York Times* published a three-generation family tree of the Bogle clan (Butterfield, 2002). It showed that Rooster had eight children, all of whom served time in prison; at the time the article appeared, two were in prison for rape, assault, robbery, and burglary. One son was in prison for murder. Although Rooster may have influenced his children to choose a life of crime, what about his four brothers? Three of them went to prison. The fourth seems to have escaped a life of crime, but of his two children, one went to prison and one was shot and killed by the police. This latter nephew of Rooster's also had two children: One committed suicide and the other is in prison. Rooster's wife has had multiple arrests, convictions, and jail sentences. Rooster also had a girlfriend who bore him two children, both of whom were in prison when the story appeared. Of 34 members of this extended family, 28 had prison records, 1 was killed by the police, 1 committed suicide, and 1 family member, a niece, had no history of arrest.

Is this a family with a strong tradition of crime, influencing younger members to take up the family business? Did Rooster and his family share a particularly pronounced genetic endowment for criminal tendencies? Did a set of genes provide a fertile ground for an active criminal enterprise? We don't have answers in the case of the Bogle clan, but evidence is emerging that helps us to disentangle the nature-nurture relationships that may pervade our lives.

A Rat Model of Early Experience, Development, and Responses to Stress

In the 1950s, Seymour Levine and his coworkers became interested in how stressful early experiences could influence the development of the endocrine and behavioral responses to stress (Levine, 1957, 2002). Using neonatal rats as their subjects, they began by separating rat pups from their mothers for varying lengths of time ranging from a few minutes to up to 24 hours. Longer periods of separation had the effect of making the animals stress hyperresponsive as adults, specific developmental stages proved more vulnerable than others, and the findings spurred research by several other groups. We will focus on some specific examples here that illustrate how early nurturing or lack of nurturing can have profound effects on gene expression, emotional and stress reactivity, and possibly health.

Maternal Separation and Neglect

After initially establishing maternal deprivation as an important event in the endocrine and behavioral development of the rat, subsequent studies indicated that maternally deprived animals were still hyperreactive to anxiety-provoking stress in adulthood. Pups that were 12 to 20 days old were separated from their mothers and kept in a warm place for 1, 8, or 24 hours before being returned to the nest (Stanton, Gutierrez, & Levine, 1988). Subsequent exposure to a novel environment showed that the animals separated for 8 and 24 hours had increasingly exaggerated corticosterone responses relative to controls, although the 1-hour deprived animals failed to show an elevation in reactivity to this stressor. Further investigation revealed that loss of maternal contact, and not simply food deprivation, was the primary source of this stress enhancement, especially for pups below 20 days of age.

Of special interest was the finding that maternal separation had a greater effect on the stress reactivity of the HPAC than on its diurnal and metabolic regulation (van Oers, de Kloet, & Levine, 1998; van Oers, de Kloet, Whelan, & Levine, 1998). Recall from Chapter 7 that the HPAC is regulated as two systems, one diurnal and metabolic and the other stress reactive. The two faces of the glucocorticoid response have different influences, with the stress-reactive response being especially dependent on hypothalamic inputs via corticotropin releasing factor (CRF) neurons from higher centers. This finding makes this an especially interesting experimental model for observing brain changes involved in emotional reactivity and responsiveness of the HPAC in particular. The stress of maternal separation acutely activates the locus ceruleus (Dent, Smith, & Levine, 2001), causing release of norepinephrine at the hypothalamic paraventricular nucleus (PVN). Recall that the locus ceruleus is the brainstem nucleus responsible for regulating global activation of the central nervous system and in part for activating the PVN. Equally important are results indicating an effect of maternal-deprivation stress on the hippocampus. Deprivation is associated with an increase in the numbers of hippocampal serotonin receptors (Vazquez, Lopez, Van Hoers, Watson, & Levine, 2000), perhaps consistent with a reduced release of serotonin and a consequent upregulation of receptor numbers.

Longer-term effects on the brain are also indicated by the fact that deprived rats have higher rates of neuron and glial cell death during early life in several brain regions (Zhang et al., 2002), including mossy fibers of the hippocampus (Huot, Thrivikraman, Meaney, & Plotsky, 2001). Because small hippocampal volume and high levels of glucocorticoids are associated with risk for depression, the effects of such early life stress may show up as psychopathology in later life. Even less severe, but more frequent, maternal deprivation, consisting of 3 hours of daily separation for 2 weeks during nursing, results in response alterations that persist into adulthood. These animals are anxiety prone as adults and are more likely to consume water that contains alcohol than are undeprived control rats (Huot et al., 2001). Such animals may also have altered central dopamine dynamics and elevated sensitivity to cocaine and amphetamine (Meaney, Brake, & Gratton, 2002).

These findings thus appear to be of critical significance in our thinking about adverse early life experiences and their effects on development of the limbic system and the stress axis more generally. A single episode of severe stress, equivalent to the pups' being abandoned for a full day, can affect development of the hippocampus, a brain region central to the regulation of the stress response and to memory formation. It is significant that these effects are specific to loss of maternal care and not to deprivation of food or warmth. Apparently, even milder deprivation has long-term effects if repeated often enough.

If severe or repeated maternal deprivation increases stress reactivity in adulthood, what aspect of nurturing is important in producing this effect? As it turns out, mothers of 24-hour-separated rats are somewhat neglectful of their duties and fail to pay much attention to their prodigal offspring when they are returned to the nest. As a result, they fail to do much licking and grooming and do not adopt a supportive nursing posture. Attempts to reverse the effects of separation have shown that manual stroking of the pups during the period of separation can avert the negative outcomes (van Oers, de Kloet, Whelan, et al., 1998). The importance of maternal licking and grooming and nursing behaviors calls attention to the potential for maternal styles to render adult offspring less stress reactive than usual.

Nurturing by Rat Mothers Is Increased by Brief Separation

Michael Meaney and his research group, in working with the maternal-separation stress model, made an interesting observation about maternal behavior and later stress reactivity of the pups. When rat pups were separated from their mothers and handled for only short periods, in this case 15 minutes per day during Days 5 to 10 of life, the adult animals were found to be stress resistant (Plotsky & Meaney, 1993). That is, when exposed to normally stressful experiences such as restraint or an open field, these animals explored more than their control counterparts and produced lower levels of corticosterone. Examination of data across studies indicated that animals separated for brief periods had increased expression of glucocorticoid receptors in both the hippocampus and frontal cortex (Liu et al., 1997; Meaney et al., 1985). Observation of the behavior of the rat mothers during these experiments proved to be revealing. When pups were separated for long periods, say 3 to 24 hours, the mothers behaved as if they had become neglectful parents. After the pups were returned to the nest, the mothers tended to ignore them or failed to counteract the stress effects with extra nurturing. The exact opposite occurred in the case of the brief 15-minute separation model. In this case, the mothers immediately gathered up their separated pups, put them into the nest, licked and groomed them, and began to nurse them using a posture that ensured the pups got the maximum amount of milk from a nursing bout.

Studies of brain differences in nurtured and control pups showed a high level of serotonin release at the hippocampus, which serves to activate transcription factors that contribute positively to expression of genes for glucocorticoid receptors (Laplante, Diorio, & Meaney, 2002; Weaver, Aherne, Meaney, Schaefer, & Dixon, 2000; Weaver, Grant, & Meaney, 2002). This altered gene expression, making these animals less stress reactive for their lifetimes. The high number of glucocorticoid receptors allows stress responses to be quickly dampened when started. Other evidence suggests lower levels of CNS CRF expression, so that activation of the stress axis is itself lower. This clear finding that a behavioral experience early in life can program genes that have a broad effect on behavioral and stress reactivity has far-reaching consequences for thinking about early experience, development, and vulnerability to certain events in later life.

This raises the question of whether the stress of brief separation of the pups from their mothers was itself a critical event or whether the 15-minute separations only served to elicit natural nurturing behaviors in the mothers. It turns out that short separations of 15 minutes are well within the norm for wild rats. The pups do not produce stress calls. So the pups may not have a direct response to the separation itself. As to maternal behaviors, careful observation reveals wide variations in spontaneous licking and grooming and other nurturing behaviors in nesting rat mothers (Liu et al., 1997). Some mothers are consistently nurturing. They spontaneously lick, groom, and nurse to a high degree, just as if the pups have been briefly separated from them. Other mothers are naturally less solicitous and are fairly casual in carrying out their maternal duties. These findings suggest that in the 15-minute separation paradigm, the maternal behaviors themselves are the crucial event. The separation serves to elicit natural maternal behaviors in the mothers, not to stress the pups. Rat pups reared by mothers who are high in licking and grooming have the same brain and behavioral changes as rats that are first separated before being licked and groomed.

We might wonder if offspring of licking and grooming mothers become stress resistant because they were born with a set of gene variations different from their casually reared counterparts. A way to test this is to do cross-fostering studies. In this case, pups are deliberately traded from one mother to another so that high-licking and grooming mothers end up rearing offspring of low-licking and grooming mothers and vice versa. If the genes that are inherited are critical, it should make little or no difference how the mothers behave; on the other hand, if the maternal behavior is crucial, the mother of origin should not affect the results. The maternal behavior turns out to be the crucial link. Regardless of whether pups are born to nurturing or nonnurturing mothers, if they are taken in by high-licking and grooming foster mothers, they prove to be stress resistant as adults, and the stress-resistant brain changes show in their rearing pattern. What turns out to be perhaps more interesting is that female pups reared by high-licking and grooming moms are also more likely to be highly nurturing when they mature and become mothers (Meaney, 2001). The fact that these second-generation mothers have high levels of serotonin activity and low CRF expression shows that the transmission of this behavioral trait is "nongenomic"—that is, based not on the genome but on the effects of the environment on the expression of genes in the genome. In this case, the crucial element in the environment is social: the behavior of the mother toward the offspring.

It is quite tempting to think of the nurturing rat mothers as good mothers and the less nurturing ones as delinquent in their duty. Similarly, it is tempting to think of the offspring of these types of mothers as better if they are "stress resistant" and worse if they are "stress prone." We should keep in mind that judging the worth of rats as mothers in this way imposes too many contemporary human values onto this situation. Similarly, the judgment implied in terms like *stress prone* reads more into the situation than is called for. Meaney (2001) himself sounded a cautionary note. Taking a more behavioral ecological view, he pointed out that brief periods of maternal separation are normal for pups born to mothers who are highly dominant and thus have nearby sources of food and water and live in relative safety. As a result, the mothers themselves are less subject to danger and daily stresses. In contrast, pups born to mothers who are less dominant and thus are far from food and water and must traverse greater dangers on a daily basis are usually left alone for long periods, and their mothers are more frequently stressed. Such pups consequently receive less care and attention. When they grow up, they are highly reactive to the environment. Perhaps this is an adaptive quality when the environment is harsh and dangerous. In fact, a placid, low-anxiety rat that was content to explore new places without fear would not last long in a dangerous world occupied by predators. So, setting the value judgments aside, we can see that the maternal behavior is, in Meaney's words, a means of intergenerational gene imprinting by the mother on the offspring. This becomes a message for a lifetime that communicates to the newborn what kind of environment to be prepared for as an adult.

That said, there are a couple of useful lessons from this work. First, stress reactivity appears to be programmable by the behavior of mothers, at least in rats, and one suspects that there must be human counterparts that show the effect of parenting on development. One human counterpart is seen in maternal behavior and infant weight gain. The nurtured rats in the above studies are higher in body weight as adults than neglected rats (Levine, 1957), and recent work with human premature babies shows that active stroking and handling improves weight gain and growth rate and dramatically reduces the hospital stay before the baby can safely go home (Dieter, Field, Hernandez-Reif, Emory, & Redzepi, 2003). Other work on human nurturing shows that when mothers use large amounts of "motherese" speech with their newborns, the babies have more rapid weight gain during the first 11 months of life than do babies whose mothers talk very little or who use mainly adult speech with the baby (Monnot, 1999).

Interestingly, interacting with an infant spontaneously evokes motherese speech in both men and women and does so among people of all cultures studied to date, even when the native language does not include the large swooping, singsong vowel sounds that characterize this form of speech. Nurturing styles therefore appear to have physiological effects on humans as well as nonhuman species. Second, nurturing styles, instead of being bad or good, may convey critical information to the developing organism about the nature of the local environment that may enhance survival and the ability to cope with environments that may be more stressful when this is called for. Third, in the rat model we have just reviewed, the means of stress reactivity programming is through environmental shaping of the gene expression by a given genome. Gene responsivity to the environment is perhaps the most far-reaching implication of this work because it indicates how deeply experience can delve into the structure and function of a developing organism. This helps us think more clearly about the nature and nurture question as it affects stress reactivity.

Genotype, Early Experience, and Psychobehavioral Outcomes

Research in rats illustrated how gene expression could vary in the offspring in relation to maternal behaviors, with differing behavioral outcomes in adulthood. The genes themselves did not differ across the nurtured and neglected animals. This nevertheless raises the question of how experiences during development affect persons who have different genetic endowments. In a sense, the Meaney experiments could be conducted on two independent groups with different genetic endowments, and the interaction between the genes and the environment could then be studied. Two recent examples are ideally suited to this question, and we will review each briefly. Both studies derive from a cohort of young adults being followed in the Dunedin Multidisciplinary Health and Development Study. The study is following 1,037 children who were born in Dunedin, New Zealand, in 1972–73 and were first assessed at the Dunedin Mulitidisciplinary Health and Development Unit when they were aged 3 years. They comprise 535 males and 502 females, 1,013 singletons and 24 twins. A total of 1,015 of these young adults are still alive in 2004. Through this well-characterized cohort, it has been possible to do a limited amount of genotyping and to examine genotype differences in relation to life experience and life outcomes into early adulthood.

The MAOA Gene and
Vulnerability to Childhood Maltreatment

In the first study of interest, Caspi et al. (2002) examined persons possessing two common variants of the gene for monoamine oxidase type A (MAOA). The monoamine neurotransmitters in the central nervous system (norepinephrine, dopamine, serotonin) are critical for regulating frontal-limbic functions and global central nervous system activation. For these transmitters to function properly—that is, to allow neurons to communicate clearly and effectively—they must be present in the synapse when needed, must be eliminated when not needed, and must thereby speak a coordinated language. This means that the release of the transmitters into the synapse must be efficient, but so must their inactivation. In the case of the monoamine transmitters, most is taken back up by the presynaptic nerve ending immediately after being released. The portion that fails to be taken up is broken down outside the neuron by MAOA. The ability of MAOA to do this job effectively determines the efficiency of the inactivation of the depolarization of the postsynaptic neuron and therefore the clarity and coordination of the messages between neurons.

The gene that codes for MAOA comes in two major variants or *alleles*. This gene is sex linked and appears on the X chromosome, so females inherit one copy from each parent, and males inherit only one copy from a single parent. The proteins made by these two alleles have slightly different chains of amino acids, and this difference accounts for a small but important difference in how effectively the resulting MAOA can break down these neurotransmitters. One variant can be referred to as being high and the other low in enzymatic activity. In a simplifying manner, we can think of low-activity MAOA as causing the aminergic regulation of the central nervous system to be less precise and perhaps less in tune with external environmental demands. In this cohort, the low-activity allele was found in 37% of the 442 males and in 12% of the 481 females, who had to inherit two low-activity copies. We might think of the 37% and 12% subgroups as being at risk for given outcomes as a function of poor central MAO function.

Along with genotyping, cohort members were assessed for antisocial behavior with a scale that took into account four indices of poor social adjustment (diagnosis of conduct disorder, diagnosis of antisocial personality disorder, proneness to violence as reported in interviews of parents and teachers, and conviction in a court of law for a violent offense). Finally, the upbringing of the cohort was examined for instances of early life stress at ages 3 to 11 years, yielding three categories of early life stress exposure: "absent," "probably present," or "present in severe form."

Examples of maltreatment included observations of harsh or uncaring behavior by the mother; frequent use of spanking as a form of discipline; changes in the adult caregiver due to divorce, death, or adoption; severe physical abuse such as spanking with a leather belt; and sexual abuse.

The question of interest was whether persons who later displayed antisocial behavior had a different combination of low-activity MAOA genes and were maltreated during childhood. The results are shown in Figures 10.1 and 10.2. Figure 10.1 indicates that the extent of antisocial behavior rose substantially among abused children, but especially in those possessing the gene variant for low-activity MAOA. If the child had the high-activity MAOA variant, the influence of maltreatment on the development of antisocial behavior was greatly diminished. Figure 10.2 presents a similar analysis with the antisocial composite divided into its four components. In each form of maltreatment, the vulnerability of the individual to its effects was enhanced by the low-activity MAOA variant and buffered by the high-activity version.

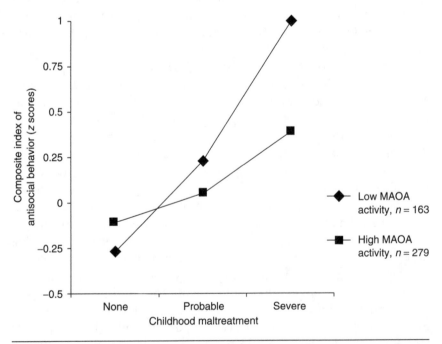

Figure 10.1   MAOA and antisocial behavior. Antisocial behavior is much more likely to emerge in persons with a history of maltreatment, but especially if they have a genetic risk factor. (Redrawn from Caspi et al., 2002.)

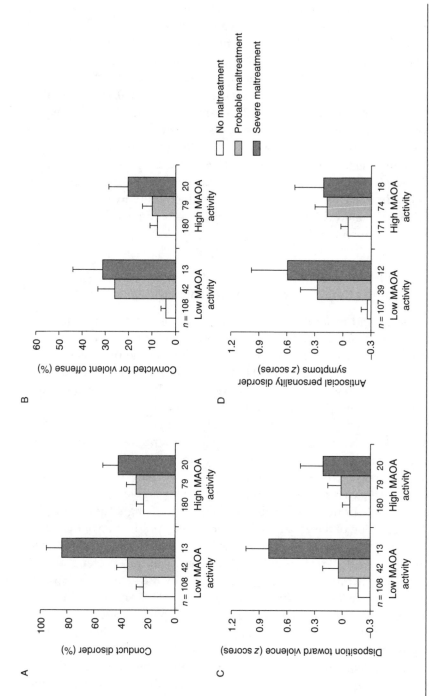

Figure 10.2 MAOA and forms of maltreatment. Several forms of maltreatment appear to result in antisocial behavior tendencies, especially in persons who possess the low-activity MAOA allele. (Redrawn from Caspi et al., 2002.)

189

Of particular interest is the percentage of males convicted of a violent offense if they had been abused and also possessed the low-activity MAOA allele. Persons with the low-activity allele who had no evidence of childhood abuse were very unlikely to have a conviction for a violent crime, whereas those who were definitely abused had a relatively high rate of 30% convictions. The relative risk, given as the Odds Ratio, showed that abused low-activity-allele persons were 9.8 times as likely to be convicted of a violent crime as their nonabused counterparts ($p < .001$). In contrast, the Odds Ratio for the high-activity-allele group was 1.63 and was not statistically significant. These results appear to show that the low-activity MAOA gene does not itself determine the outcome for these children. It does appear to confer a vulnerability to adversity, such that the maltreated children are more likely to become antisocial and to commit violent crimes.

The Serotonin Transporter Gene and Vulnerability to Childhood Maltreatment

In the second example of genes, childhood experience, and life outcome, we turn again to the Dunedin cohort study. In this case, Caspi and his coworkers were interested in how variations in the promoter region for the serotonin transporter (5-HTT) gene would be related to vulnerability to maltreatment and life stressors, with risk for depression as the outcome of interest (Caspi et al., 2003). Serotonin (5-hydroxytryptophane, or 5-HT for short) is an important regulatory neurotransmitter, as discussed in Chapter 6. The 5-HTT gene codes for a protein that transports 5-HT from the synapse back into the presynaptic terminal in order to regulate serotonin-mediated neurotransmission. A gene promoter region determines the ease of expression of the gene for a given protein. In this case, one allele of the 5-HTT promoter region (the long allele) allows for ready expression of the gene and therefore ease of production of the transporter molecule itself. The short allele determines low levels of transporter production. Bear in mind that the quantity of transporter protein a neuron manufactures will determine how readily the neuron can have its synaptic activity reduced by uptake of the 5-HT transmitter into the presynaptic terminal. If transporter levels and synaptic reuptake determine 5-HT patterning in the brain, we might expect that high levels of transporter will predict better frontal-limbic function than low levels. Does this translate into differential vulnerability to life experience?

The 5-HTT gene is autosomal, so everyone inherits two copies, one from each parent. Persons possessing the long/long allele combination have about two times the serotonin reuptake activity of those with a long/short or a short/short combination. Caspi classified genetic vulnerability into three groups: low (long/long, $n = 265$), medium (long/short, $n = 435$), and high (short/short, $n = 147$), with males and females occurring in equal proportions in each risk group. Childhood maltreatment was documented as in the previous study, and in addition, the number of stressful life events was noted for the 5 years from ages 21 to 26 years. Stressors included unemployment, financial problems, being homeless or moving often, and health or relationship problems. The results are given in Figures 10.3 and 10.4.

The effect of numbers of stressful life events on persons at the three levels of vulnerability to diagnosis or other signs of depression is shown in Figure 10.3. Two things stand out in this analysis. First, for all four depression indicators, the presence of the short allele seems to have a graded, or dose-response, relationship to adverse life events in determining the severity of the given indicator. Risk of suicide is especially striking here. In Figure 10.4, we can see the likelihood of depressive episodes in persons with three degrees of maltreatment as a child. Again, there is a well-graded relationship between severity of maltreatment and depressive episodes with the short/short allele group being most vulnerable.

The overall shape of these findings concerning the 5-HTT gene is strikingly similar to those concerning the MAOA gene. In both cases, the presence of a gene coding for less effective frontal-limbic neurochemical functioning renders an individual vulnerable to adversity in life, with childhood maltreatment being an especially negative indicator of future well-being. These results have a positive side as well. Persons with the allele variants that code for suspected better functioning are in fact resistant to the insults that life may throw their way. We may think of them as stress-hardy, or resilient, individuals.

Discussion

One wonders if the members of the Bogle clan possess a gene variant that renders their behavior more risk taking, less subject to social restraint, and less empathetic toward others and that consequently the children grow up to be risk takers with no concern for others. In choosing mates, do they find others like themselves? We don't know.

On somewhat firmer ground, the research examples I chose to present here are the best ones I have found to illustrate the interactions between a person's genes and the environment, particularly the social environment,

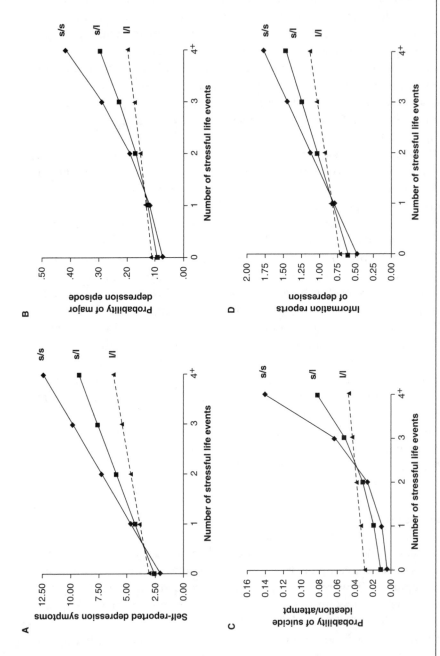

Figure 10.3 Serotonin transporter gene and stressful life events. Persons having low-efficiency production of the serotonin transporter molecule are vulnerable to depression following negative life events. (Redrawn from Caspi et al., 2002.)

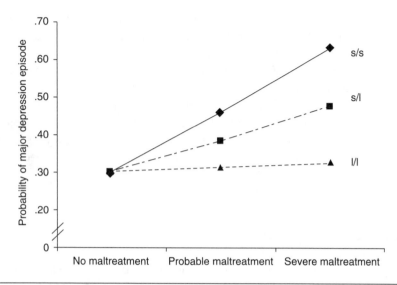

Figure 10.4   Serotonin transporter gene and childhood maltreatment. Persons having low-efficiency production of the serotonin transporter molecule (s/s) are vulnerable to depression if they were maltreated as children. Persons with the normal allele (l/l) appear somewhat resistant to the effects of maltreatment. (Redrawn from Caspi et al., 2003.)

and particularly events earlier rather than later in life. I have also chosen them because it is my guess that these will stand as paradigms for a great deal of work to come. In fact, *Science* magazine selected the Caspi work as the second most important breakthrough in all fields of science for the year 2003. (The outright winner was a breakthrough in cosmology that established the prevalence of dark matter and the developing shape of the universe.) These models, including the work of Levine, Meaney and Caspi, all illustrate that stressful events, characterized by limited control and threat to well-being, are powerful shapers of our development. They determine what appear to be lifelong trajectories for the affected individuals. The role of genes is clearly critical here, whether it is the activation of genes by other messengers or the actual presence of a given gene variant. The genes are clearly interacting with the environment, and a benign, nurturing upbringing is clearly a stimulus powerfully different from a harsh and stressful one.

The studies by Caspi are examples of gene programming. The expression of a given genome is programmed by life experience. A related example of the effect of early life stress, in this case on metabolic processes and global health in later life, is from work on the adult offspring of women exposed to severe malnutrition during pregnancy at the end of World War II in Holland. These women gave birth to low-birth-weight infants who showed elevated risk of coronary artery disease, hypertension, and premature death (Barker, 1990; Roseboom et al., 2001). The implications are that early experience of severe stress can be far reaching and can influence not only behavior but also health throughout a person's life. In relation to our present topic of stress and health, studies such as these tell us some places to look for the source of individual differences in stress reactivity, the topic of Chapter 11.

Summary

This chapter addresses a significant emerging topic in the field of stress research. Although we have long known that stress does not affect all persons equally, the full nature of the differential susceptibility to stress was unclear. The studies here suggest two basic sets of relationships. First, environmental influences can create neural signals that affect the development of the nervous system, potentially increasing gene expression or decreasing it, to produce permanent effects in the emotionality and stress reactivity of the affected individual. These neural effects may alter the stress proneness and overall health of the person through the life span. The second model is that a person may inherit a given gene variant that can affect how the person responds to stress or nurturing, again with an influence through the person's life. Neither model supports an idea that the genes themselves dictate a given outcome. In fact, the genes appear to depend on the environment to have their full expression. This gene-environment interaction provides powerful insights into the nature-nurture debate. Undoubtedly a great deal more will be discovered using both examples.

Further Reading

Levine, S. (2002). Influence of psychological variables on the activity of the hypothalamic-pituitary-adrenal axis. *European Journal of Pharmacology, 405,* 149–160.

A brief overview of the research on stress and maternal behavior on glucocorticoid reactivity to stress.

Meaney, M. J. (2001). Maternal care, gene expression, and the transmission of individual differences in stress reactivity across generations. *Annual Review of Neuroscience, 24,* 1161–1192.

An excellent overview of the author's work and that of his predecessors on the long-term effects of maternal behavior on gene expression affecting the stress axis and the transmissibility of maternal behavioral tendencies.

Monnot, M. (1999). Function of infant-directed speech. *Human Nature: An Interdisciplinary Biosocial Perspective, 10,* 415–443.

A description of the initial study of motherese speech and infant growth and development.

Pinker, S. (2002). *The blank slate: The modern denial of human nature.* New York: Viking.

An engaging, sometimes contentious, discussion of the nature-nurture controversy as it regards the gene-versus-environment dichotomy, with an engaging look at numerous aspects of child development by one of the foremost experts on language acquisition.

11

Individual Differences in Reactivity to Stress

W e have all seen how differently people respond to stress, not just in their initial reactions, but also in their ability to cope, and even in their physiological responses. We might say that the subject of individual differences is what makes the study of stress so interesting. This chapter will discuss some ways to divide the topic of stress reactivity that will help organize results of existing research and potentially identify gaps in our knowledge. To organize our discussion of individual differences in stress reactivity, we will draw on the material in Chapters 6, 7, and 10. Using the model that physiological functioning has a layered hierarchy of controls, we will describe three major sources of individual differences in reactivity to psychological stressors: (a) Persons may differ because of their cognitive and emotional characteristics, reflecting operation of frontal-limbic processes on patterns of response; (b) they may have exaggerated autonomic and endocrine responses because of differential activation of hypothalamic and brainstem outputs; and (c) they may have altered peripheral responses that reflect changes in the tissues themselves. Finally, we will consider implications of these sources of individual differences for health and disease.

The idea that our physiological dispositions and responses are tied to our state of health and risk for disease is not new. The Greeks held to a humoral theory, based on the idea that the balance of our vital humors determined how the environment affected us—an idea maintained in our everyday speech, as in "He's under the weather today." The humors also determined our pattern of disease susceptibility. We could certainly call this an early form of a *reactivity hypothesis,* one that specified differences between people in personality or temperament, physiological reactivity, and disease risk. The most prominent modern statement of an explicit reactivity hypothesis and its prediction of disease was in a paper by Hines and Brown (1932). These physician researchers advanced the idea that the size of the blood pressure response to a specific stressor (placing a hand or foot into ice water for 60 to 90 seconds) could indicate the likelihood that the person would later develop hypertension. In a more modern context, physicians commonly use stressor challenges to test the integrity of a system. For example, if a doctor suspects that a patient has diabetes, it is typical to perform a glucose tolerance test. The patient drinks a glucose and water mixture, and blood is sampled to test for the secretion of insulin and the time course of this response. A departure from the normal pattern is an indication of incorrect response to and handling of the glucose load. In turn, this information informs a diagnosis or dictates other tests. In this case, the departure in reactivity pattern from normal is considered an index of existing disease. In the field of behavioral medicine, many researchers maintain that exaggerated responses to stress act either to cause disease or to aggravate existing disease and that reducing reactivity can alleviate or prevent disease. There appears to be increasing evidence that this is so. This area has been extensively reviewed in a series of recent papers (Kamarck & Lovallo, 2003; Linden, Gerin, & Davidson, 2003; Lovallo & Gerin, 2003; Schwartz et al., 2003; Treiber et al., 2003).

Persons May Differ in Stress Reactivity Because of Inborn Factors or Experience

As we noted in Chapter 10, experience may have a lasting effect on responses to stressors. Michael Meaney's work clearly demonstrates that maternal nurturing in rats can increase serotonin activity and reduce glucocorticoid responsiveness throughout life. On the other hand, Levine's and Nemeroff's work shows that repeated or severe stress early in life has deleterious effects on the animal's responsiveness. In both cases, the reactive tendency of the central nervous system has been shifted by the early life experience. In addition to the role of experience, we know that genetic factors can determine differences in psychological and physiological responses to stress. The clearest evidence of inborn differences in stress response comes from studies of the spontaneously hypertensive rat, an animal that is hyperreactive both behaviorally and physiologically

(Knardahl & Hendley, 1990). Similarly, monkeys from the same species raised in identical circumstances still show large individual differences in heart rate responses to behavioral threats as well as in aggressiveness and affiliative tendencies (Kaplan, Manuck, Clarkson, & Prichard, 1985). The work summarized in Chapter 10 on genes, experience, and health outcomes alerts us to the ways that our genetic endowment and our life experience interact in determining our characteristic ways of reacting to challenges in daily life. To reduce this complexity, I have found it helpful in my own thinking about individual differences to consider the organization of our central nervous system and peripheral response systems at three somewhat separable levels. We will discuss these and present some data suggesting that the three-level approach is useful in interpreting studies of health outcomes.

Individual Differences in Stress Responses May Be Determined by Functional Alterations at Three Levels in the System

There are potentially three levels at which persons may differ in how they react to threats. These levels correspond to major components of our model of central nervous system functioning in Chapter 6, and these are summarized in Figure 11.1.

First, at the top level of organization, persons may differ in *frontal-limbic activity* in relation to their primary appraisals of events and their secondary appraisals of available coping resources, on the basis of personal experiences, stored as declarative memories, and due to emotion-based reactions arising from conditioned associations. These processes correspond to activities associated with cognitive evaluations in working memory and with the affective biasing of these evaluations that is necessary for making decisions. These decision-making functions are associated with the prefrontal cortex working in light of inputs from the limbic system. The limbic inputs arise in particular from the amygdala and bed nucleus of the stria terminalis and their actions on subcortical nuclei that interact with the prefrontal cortex.

Second, evaluations and emotions shaped by these higher-level processes act on the hypothalamus and brainstem. Hypothalamic areas such as the HACER and paraventricular nucleus may consistently be more or less reactive to a given set of messages from the higher areas. These gain factors may determine the responsiveness of the hypothalamus to descending activation, and this may constitute a consistent source

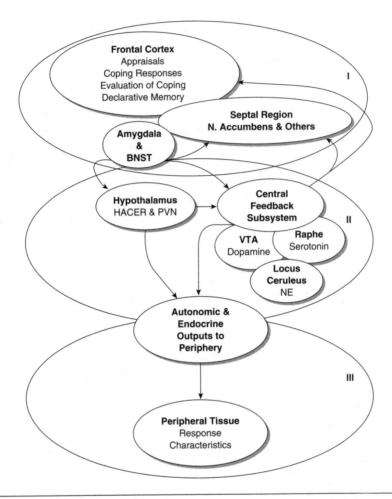

Figure 11.1   Three levels of control over stress reactivity. I. Individual differences in reaction to threats from the environment may occur as the outcome of frontal-limbic processes. These bring together the actions of working memory, declarative memories, and Pavlovian conditioning and are shaped by inputs from the amygdala and the central feedback subsystem. This level of reactivity shaping appears clearly in subjects' self-reports, subjective experience, and psychological or temperament-based personal characteristics. II. Persons may differ in the reactive tendency of the hypothalamus, especially the paraventricular nucleus and the area identified as the HACER. At this same level of analysis, differences in outputs to frontal-limbic areas from the aminergic brainstem nuclei that constitute the central feedback subsystem will also shape individual differences in reactivity. They exert an affective bias on the frontal-limbic areas, and they affect descending activity in autonomic pathways. III. Peripheral organs may function differently in different persons and therefore have different patterns and degrees of response for any given output from the hypothalamus and brainstem.

of differences between persons in how they respond to stress. In similar fashion, brainstem aminergic nuclei may contribute to interpersonal reactivity differences in two ways: (a) The aminergic nuclei may differ from person to person in the strength and patterning of the signals they return to the rest of the central nervous system; and (b) the descending outputs of these brainstem nuclei may similarly differ in the strength of their outputs to the peripheral organs via the intermediolateral cell column and the nucleus of the solitary tract.

Third, peripheral organs may be more or less responsive to the signals they receive. They may have different complements of autonomic receptors, they may be genetically prone to disease, and both of these factors may determine that peripheral responsivity is altered from normal.

Individual Differences in Evaluative and Emotional Processes

The top level of the diagram in Figure 11.1 concerns brain areas specialized for shaping our evaluations and associated emotional responses to events, processes we associate with primary and secondary appraisals. Several lines of evidence suggest that there may be stable differences between persons in the formation of situational judgments and the development of the emotions that accompany them. On the basis of personal experience, we recognize the pervasiveness of declarative memories and Pavlovian conditioned responses and how we use these to help us classify events and choose responses to them, especially if they are threats to our well-being. The second line of evidence comes from work on temperament differences, affective response differences, and accompanying physiological differences in response to specific challenges. In both cases, there are neurophysiological mechanisms that generate descending signals to the hypothalamus and brainstem and cause responses in the periphery.

Neurophysiological Evidence on Prefrontal-Limbic Connections and Emotions

In Lazarus and Folkman's (1984) model of appraisals and coping, we think first of how cognitive evaluations occur in working memory and how these deliberations are informed by experiences maintained in declarative memory, and we consider that these functions depend on activities of the prefrontal cortex. Because we each differ in our life experience, we are likely to differ in how we interpret events and how we form emotions in relation to these interpretations. Interpretation of events and their evaluation based on experience occur in working memory. Work by Goldman-Rakic (reviewed in Ungerleider, 1995) shows that areas of the dorsolateral prefrontal cortex are differentially activated during tasks requiring working memory. These cortical areas are tied to the architecture of sensory systems and are accessible to declarative (long-term) memory. This allows the prefrontal cortex to have the benefit of prior experience while processing current inputs. However, we know that declarative and working memory alone do not allow normal, adaptive decision making. These areas also need inputs from areas of the brain that we usually associate with the emotions (Damasio, 1994). For our decision making to benefit from the affective biasing that must occur for us to make useful decisions, we also need inputs from limbic structures, especially the amygdala, acting on frontal-limbic circuits, such as those referenced in Figure 6.8. These limbic inputs are shaped by other aspects of experience, especially the motivational or affective components of our experience that we retain through Pavlovian conditioning.

In a similar line of reasoning, LeDoux (1993) considers the hippocampus to be critical for the recall of specific events in our lives and the amygdala to be essential for recall of the contextual aspects of these events through its role in Pavlovian conditioning. We may therefore think of working memory as the highest venue for integrating our past with our present via declarative memories and Pavlovian associations. We can then invest our present experience with the benefit of our emotional evaluations. These joint influences of experience on working memory suggest that stable, but not fixed, differences between persons may be formed by life experiences that in turn may alter the evaluation of current events and the bodily outputs associated with them. These processes fall into the province of our individual psychology, but they cannot be divorced from the brain systems involved, and in the context of our discussion of reactivity, we will say that frontal-limbic processes instantiate the ground for the action of our affective-experiential response biases. Not only do these frontal-limbic processes shape our responses, but they are accessible to consciousness, and they give rise to subjective experiences that we can communicate.

A closely related approach to this topic is a model by Jeffrey Gray (1987, 1991). In bringing together cognitive and emotional components of current experience as determinants of outputs to the body, Gray proposed two distinct frontal-limbic systems responsible for interpretation of incoming events and formulation of responses. One is the *behavioral inhibition system*, thought to play a central role in fear and anxiety. This system organizes autonomic and behavioral responses to aversive conditioned stimuli. In animals, the freezing response forms a complete behavioral complex including immobility, heightened attention, and motor preparedness in the face of threat. It has been viewed as a behavioral pattern that forms a preparation for the active component of the fight-or-flight response. Gray also postulates a *behavioral approach* system that responds to appetitive events and is linked to positive emotions. Its activities serve to motivate exploration and appetitive approach behaviors. Gray's system incorporates activities of the septal nuclei. To briefly review points raised in Chapter 6, the septal nuclei include the nucleus accumbens and related structures found at the base of the ventromedial prefrontal cortex and at the rostral tip of the hypothalamus. These nuclei have inputs from the hippocampus and the amygdala along with fibers that ascend from brainstem aminergic nuclei. These brainstem nuclei support global activation (the locus ceruleus) and provide affective coloration to events that are being appraised (the raphe nuclei). They also serve to motivate approach and avoidance behaviors and to sustain attention to relevant cues (the ventral tegmental and nigro-striatal dopaminergic pathways). The aminergic nuclei themselves have inputs from the amygdala and frontal cortex, so they are key players in the frontal-limbic loops essential for evaluation of events in working memory or through less conscious processes. They therefore aid in selection of appropriate responses. These connections at the septal region were the ones specifically damaged in the case of Phineas Gage.

Not surprisingly, researchers interested in how persons differ in affective temperament are concerned with the organization of these frontal-limbic systems. Cacioppo and Berntson (1994) suggested that Gray's approach and withdrawal systems are differentially distributed in the left and right hemispheres, respectively. They argued that negative emotions associated with stressful events are differentially activated by right hemisphere structures. Given that prior experience will affect both memories and conditioned responses to situations, the behavioral approach and inhibition systems can act to motivate both behaviors and physiological responses in conjunction with primary and secondary appraisals. Richard Davidson and colleagues have observed individual differences in the asymmetry of electroencephalographic (EEG) activity measured over the left and right frontal cortex (Tomarken, Davidson, Wheeler, & Doss, 1992). Persons with greater activation of left frontal regions tend to react positively to many situations and to be highly resistant to depression. Conversely, persons with greater right-sided activation are prone to negative mood states and depressive episodes. Work by others has shown that depressed individuals have reduced metabolic activity in the left prefrontal cortex. This *modulation asymmetry* appears to be an important determinant of individual differences in emotional experience, and it appears to form a stable, traitlike characteristic. For example, shy, inhibited children are low in left frontal alpha EEG activation, and shyness is one of the most persistent emotional-behavioral traits. Adults show long-term consistency in resting alpha asymmetry and in their accompanying emotional dispositions. Right and left frontal EEG activity varies as a function of exposure to negative and positive events, respectively, and in relation to the negative and positive emotions accompanying those events. Diazepam, a potent antianxiety drug that acts on brainstem aminergic nuclei, increases approach behavior and increases left frontal activation in rhesus monkeys. Infants with greater right-sided frontal asymmetry not only experience greater negative affect but secrete more cortisol, tonically and in response to acute stress (Buss et al., 2003). Monkeys with similar frontal asymmetries are higher in fearful behavior and in cortisol activity (Kalin, Larson, Shelton, & Davidson, 1998). Soufer et al. (1998) have observed asymmetric EEG activation in heart disease patients during acute mental stress. On the basis of these results, we might expect healthy adults who differ in their left-right balance of frontal EEG asymmetries to also differ in autonomic and endocrine reactions to events associated with negative affect.

This research provides us with a neurophysiologically based view of how people differ in the shaping of their evaluative processes, emotional responses, and response choices. This view helps us appreciate that there are persistent neurophysiological differences between persons underlying their characteristic outlooks and moods and resulting physiological reactivity. These differences are almost surely a combination of inborn tendencies and life experiences. We have already noted in Chapter 10 research by Michael Meaney showing that rats developed long-term elevations in serotonergic function and became stress hyporeactive on the basis of repeated tactile stimulation and nurturing early in life. In contrast, serotonin deficiencies can result from early neglect, and these deficiencies are related to negative moods, aggression, and lack of social affiliation. The neurophysiology of affective experience has been reviewed from within this perspective by Davidson (2003).

Personality Dispositions, Emotions, and Responses to Stress

If persons differ neurophysiologically in ways that affect personality dispositions and evaluative tendencies, our model of psychological stress in Chapter 6 would lead us to expect parallel differences in how people engage their hypothalamic and brainstem areas controlling peripheral activation. Persons who have strong emotion traits tend to act these out in their overt behavior and, we suspect, in their physiological responses. As a shorthand, we refer to individual differences of this sort as *cognitive-emotional*. Persons who see the world differently from others and who have emotion response biases will have corresponding physiological response biases. We can take some examples from research on hostile and nonhostile individuals.

Suarez and Williams (1989) have shown that persons high in cynical hostility, as measured by self-reports on the Cook-Medley (Hostility) Ho scale, produce larger blood pressure responses to a task performed immediately after a social encounter with a rude laboratory assistant. Observations from a related study by Susan Everson and colleagues illustrate how social cues can trigger specific evaluations in hostility-prone persons and how these can alter physiological responses (Everson, McKey, & Lovallo, 1995). Everson interviewed the subjects to assess their potential for interpersonal hostility and invited the most and least hostile men back to the laboratory for a second, ostensibly unrelated experiment, to measure "how blood pressure was affected by mental challenges." Each person worked on two identically difficult mental arithmetic tasks separated by a 20-minute rest. The first task was done under neutral conditions for all subjects. This provided a simple baseline of reactivity to an activating but not particularly distressing task. In the second task, one third of the subjects again performed under neutral conditions to control for adaptation to repetition of the task. The other subjects were harassed during the rest period and second task to compare the reactions of the low- and high-hostile groups.

At the end of the rest interval, a new, female experimenter entered the testing room and rudely announced that the original experimenter had forgotten a prior appointment and that she would now have to finish the testing, conveying a sense of irritation at this inconvenience. She removed the subject's magazines just as a phone outside the door rang. She then held a staged conversation, gossiping about friends' hairdos and dating habits, at last remarking in a bored voice that she had to "finish up with this guy in here." She then made several gratuitous harassing comments during the second task.

The subjects' reports give us insight into differences in how the high- and low-hostile men saw the interpersonal dynamics of the social situation. First, one high-hostile subject became irate and announced that he would not participate in a study conducted by such rude and uncaring people! (Naturally, he was debriefed and told about the purpose of the study, as were all subjects.) Second, high-hostile men more often said they felt that the experimenter was directing her callous attitude toward them personally, while low-hostile men often imagined that the new experimenter was merely having a bad day. These reports indicate an important difference in the groups' primary appraisals of the situation. Third, when questioned about their suspicions, about twice as many low-hostile as high-hostile men had doubts about the validity of the scenario. It was as if the less hostile men could calmly reflect on the situation whereas high-hostile men were prepared to react from a hostile standpoint and reacted without reflection. Structured mood reports indicated that high-hostile men felt more global activation and a greater sense of distress than the low-hostile men.

Along with these appraisal differences, the high- and low-hostile men also responded to the second task with different levels of cardiovascular activation. Figure 11.2 shows the response differences from the first to the second tasks for harassment and the control condition. The high-hostile men had consistently greater responses to the second task in the harassment condition. The *rate pressure product* (heart rate multiplied by systolic blood pressure) is a simple measure of oxygen demand by the heart muscle that indexes the workload the heart is under at the time of measurement. The responses of the harassed subjects did not diminish to the second task, and in fact they increased for the highly hostile subjects. In contrast, the low-hostile group and the control subjects, who were not harassed, both had lower levels of cardiovascular function during the second mental arithmetic task.

The high-hostile subjects apparently evaluated the situation within a hostile cognitive scheme, became offended and angry, and then produced high levels of sympathetically mediated cardiovascular activity. We speculate that these autonomic response differences were derived ultimately from emotion-related differences in frontal-limbic processing of the harassment. These in turn may have resulted in greater hypothalamic activation and therefore responses of brainstem cardiovascular control centers. This is consistent with results in hostile subjects showing greater reduction of vagal control of the heart in response to psychological challenges but not physical ones such as orthostatic testing (Sloan et al., 2001).

Other work of this sort shows that highly hostile male subjects who are harassed during work on an anagram task have larger and more prolonged activation of cardiovascular, catecholamine, and cortisol responses (Suarez, Kuhn, Schanberg, Williams, & Zimmermann, 1998). Hostility is associated with altered beta-adrenergic activation consistent with more pronounced blood pressure rises to aggravating challenge (Hughes, Sherwood, Blumenthal, Suarez, & Hinderliter, 2003). Still other work shows that habitual differences in hostility may relate

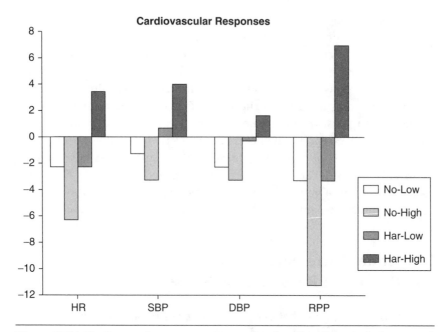

Figure 11.2 Cardiovascular responses to a mental arithmetic task under neutral conditions and conditions of harassment (Har) for high- and low-hostile men. Bars show responses relative to the responses to an earlier task administered under non-harassing conditions. Note that only the high-hostile men consistently produced larger responses to the harassment. HR = heart rate, SBP = systolic blood pressure, DBP = diastolic blood pressure, RPP = rate pressure product. (Redrawn from Everson et al., 1995.)

to slower metabolism of triglycerides, suggesting longer periods of blood lipid elevation after a fatty meal (Engbretson & Stoney, 1993), and with altered immune system function (Suarez, 2003). This indicates that hostile biases in situational evaluations and resulting emotions may predict health-related alterations in such health indicators as lipoprotein transport and immune system function. These provide further evidence converging with earlier findings that hostility is an independent predictor of premature death due to heart attack and other forms of sudden death (Dembroski, MacDougall, Costa, & Grandits, 1989). In relation to our cognitive-emotional interpretation, persons who ruminate about prior stressors have prolonged activation of cardiovascular function (Glynn, Christenfeld, & Gerin, 2002). Schwartz et al. (2003) argued that rumination about emotionally charged events may contribute to the total health burden of increased reactivity.

In this section, we focused on persons who manifest hostile traits exposed to hostility provocations in the lab. The studies suggest that the high-hostile subjects were primed to draw hostile interpretations of social interactions, with resulting differences in their emotional reactions. We believe these were accompanied by different frontal-limbic response patterns resulting in disproportionate effects on the hypothalamus and brainstem outputs to autonomic and endocrine pathways. In the next section, we will consider whether there are individual differences in stress reactivity that do not depend on these kinds of differences in situational appraisals or lack of coping resources. Exaggerated stress reactivity of this sort would point away from frontal-limbic processes and toward hypothalamic and brainstem sources of individual differences in reactivity.

Individual Differences in Hypothalamic and Brainstem Responses to Stress

There is other evidence that persons who have similar emotional response tendencies nevertheless respond differently to stress, and we suspect that these individual differences may be hypothalamic or brainstem in origin. Research on cardiovascular reactivity provides us with examples of persons who have quite elevated cardiovascular and endocrine responses to various challenges, but they may not report feeling different about the situations they are exposed to. As a result, there is no obvious basis for saying that cognitive-emotional interpretations caused these high- and low-reactive persons to differ. We might therefore ask if it is reasonable to look at the hypothalamus and brainstem as sources of these individual differences.

Cardiovascular Reactivity

There are considerable individual differences in the magnitude of heart rate change to mentally demanding tasks, leading to speculation that persons having consistently larger responses may be at higher risk of coronary artery disease and hypertension (Sherwood & Turner, 1992). Manuck and Garland (1980) found that persons who had large heart rate rises to a cognitively challenging task had similarly large responses to the same task and to a different cognitive task when retested 13 months later. Others have reported reasonably high levels of reactivity over 10 years (Sherwood et al., 1997). This made it possible to consider heart rate reactivity a stable individual difference, somewhat like a personality trait.

Heart rate reactivity is also stable across different types of tasks, such as cold pressor and reaction-time tests conducted 2 weeks to 13 months apart (Lovallo, Pincomb, & Wilson, 1986a) and across public speaking and mental arithmetic tasks 3 weeks apart (Sgoutas-Emch et al., 1994), again reinforcing its traitlike qualities. This stability over time and across situations provides a basis for us to consider reactivity tendencies as capable of affecting health. The idea that persistently large cardiovascular responses may themselves be a disease risk is known as the *cardiovascular reactivity hypothesis.*

Persons who tend to respond to stress with relatively large heart rate and blood pressure increases appear to have elevated levels of sympathetic outflow from brainstem cardiovascular control centers. We discussed autonomic controls on cardiovascular function in Chapters 4 and 5. Cacioppo and colleagues provide an extensive account of measures reflecting sympathetic and parasympathetic influences on the heart (Berntson, Cacioppo, & Quigley, 1993, 1994; Cacioppo & Berntson, 1994; Cacioppo et al., 1994).

In considering the possible sources of individual differences in heart rate reactivity, we may refer to Figure 6.7. Persons who are more reactive could be more responsive at the level of the brainstem cardiovascular control nuclei, the paraventricular nucleus of the hypothalamus, or the HACER. We do not currently have strong evidence allowing us to separate these sources of differences in response magnitude. However, there are reasons to speculate that differences in heart rate reactivity arise at the level of the hypothalamus.

My colleagues and I tested subjects using a painful cold pressor test to stimulate responses to form a heart rate reactivity classification, and we also tested these subjects on reaction-time tasks using either threat of electric shock or monetary rewards as motivation (Lovallo et al., 1986a, 1986b). These studies showed that persons who had large heart rate increases (>19 beats per minute) to the cold pressor test also had the largest heart rate changes to the reaction-time tasks, regardless of the nature of the incentive. Most important for our present discussion, the heart rate reactivity groups did not differ in their perceptions or evaluations of the tasks. Overall, subjects in the shock avoidance study rated that task as much more aversive than the other subjects rated the rewarded task. However, within each study, the high heart rate reactors did not report feeling either more activated or distressed than their less reactive counterparts during either task (Lovallo, Pincomb, Brackett, & Wilson, 1990).

Because the heart rate response groups did not have different subjective experiences, we suspect that their cardiovascular response differences did not result from processes at the cognitive-emotional level in Figure 11.1. Instead, it appears that the response difference was based on activational differences lower in the system. This interpretation is consistent with findings in borderline hypertensives compared with controls at low risk of future hypertension (al'Absi et al., 1994). The borderlines had larger cortisol and cardiovascular responses to nonaversive mental stressors, with no difference in reported feelings of activation or distress, suggesting greater hypothalamic activation as the source of the reactivity difference.

Integrated Cardiac and Endocrine Reactivity

My colleagues and I reexamined the data from our studies using aversive and rewarded versions of the reaction-time task for evidence of the relationship between heart rate reactivity and cortisol responses (Lovallo et al., 1990). We compared cortisol and norepinephrine responses in high- and low–heart rate–reactive men during the two versions of the task in a combined analysis. We expected to see greater norepinephrine responses in high–heart rate reactors to both tasks and to see greater cortisol responses in this group, but only to the aversive tasks. This prediction was based on a theory that cortisol is secreted in preferentially aversive situations evoking negative emotions (Lundberg & Frankenhaeuser, 1980).

The data are displayed in Figure 11.3. First, we found that the low–heart rate reactors showed little or no change in either cortisol or norepinephrine to either task. Second, the high–heart rate reactors produced significant cortisol rises to the aversive task but not to the rewarded task. They also had larger norepinephrine responses to both tasks, indicating greater global sympathetic activation. Therefore, the tendency to produce large sympathetically mediated cardiac responses appears tied to cortisol activation under conditions evoking negative emotions.

One implication of this result is that cardiovascular reactivity may relate mechanistically to adrenocortical reactivity and therefore to modulation of the immune system. Cacioppo and colleagues have similarly shown that high–heart rate reactors produce larger cortisol responses to mental arithmetic stress (Sgoutas-Emch et al., 1994). Schommer and colleagues (Schommer, Hellhammer, & Kirschbaum, 2003) have tracked this parallel activity of the cardiovascular and endocrine systems over repeated stress episodes. A second implication is that negative mood states of any given magnitude would have a larger influence in highly reactive persons and a smaller influence in less reactive ones because of differences in a hypothesized hypothalamic gain factor.

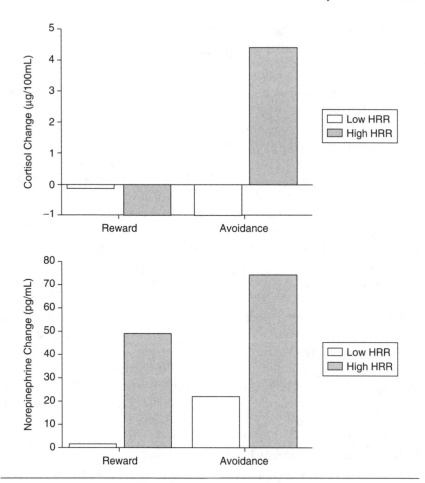

Figure 11.3   Cortisol and norepinephrine responses to reaction-time tasks under conditions of reward or shock avoidance in men known to be high or low in heart rate reactivity (HRR). The high reactors had greater norepinephrine responses to both tasks, indicating greater overall sympathetic activation. The high–heart rate reactors also had greater cortisol responses to the aversive task, indicating an association between heart rate reactivity and cortisol reactivity to conditions favoring cortisol secretion, such as the aversive task. (Redrawn from Lovallo et al., 1990.)

These results show that physiologically reactive persons may produce integrated patterns of both sympathetic and pituitary-adrenal activation. This suggests that the basis of this elevated reactivity must be integrated at a level higher than the brainstem and pituitary. The paraventricular nucleus of the hypothalamus is an ideal candidate, as is the HACER.

Central Nervous System Activity in Relation
to Cardiovascular and Endocrine Reactivity

The studies reviewed above resulted in two major conclusions. First, high– and low–heart rate reactors appear to experience challenging events in the same way, suggesting that they are not differentially reactive because of differences in evaluations of the situation or the resulting emotions. Second, the tendency for large heart rate responses to be accompanied by large cortisol responses suggests that this individual difference in stress reactivity is organized at a level above the separate output pathways for autonomic and endocrine outflow. This leads us to focus on the hypothalamus as the structure most capable of producing this integrated response pattern. Whether the difference is at the level of the HACER or portions of the hypothalamus that communicate more directly with the pituitary and brainstem, such as the paraventricular nucleus, is not clear from these data, but the pattern of results is consistent with a focus on the hypothalamus.

This line of reasoning leads to the picture of differences in heart rate reactivity that result from individual differences in the *hypothalamic amplification* of signals arriving from evaluative and emotion-producing centers of the brain. The presumed amplification difference may therefore result in consistent individual differences in integrated autonomic and endocrine outflow, accounting for the differences between subjects in both heart rate and cortisol responses. Although the case for differences in hypothalamic amplification of descending signals is indirect, there is a plausible mechanism for such a system in limbic and hypothalamic outputs. As noted in Chapter 7, high levels of cortisol exposure can sensitize the amygdala and consequently exaggerate CRF neuron inputs to the PVN and HACER during times of stress (Schulkin et al., 1998; Shepard et al., 2000, 2003). More direct evidence has emerged from a study of humans who died with complications of hypertension. In the deceased hypertensive patients, the number of CRF neurons in the hypothalamic PVN was greater than in control autopsy tissue (Goncharuk, Van Heerikhuize, Swaab, & Buijs, 2002). According to the researchers, "Increased activity of CRH-producing neurons in the PVN of hypertensive patients is proposed not only to entail hyperactivity of the hypothalamo-pituitary-adrenal axis, but also of the sympathetic nervous system and, thus, to be involved in the pathogenesis of hypertension" (p. 321). In relation to our present discussion, such persons would have larger cardiovascular and endocrine responses to a variety of stressors regardless of their individual cognitive-emotional reactions.

Individual Differences in Peripheral Responses to Stress

At the peripheral level, abnormal stress responses are recognized as signs of existing disease. In endocrinology, for example, failure to remove glucose from the blood following glucose challenge may indicate diabetes. In cardiology, premature fatigue, shortness of breath, exaggerated blood pressure response, or abnormal cardiac rhythm during exercise stress signals the presence of coronary artery disease, hypertension, or autonomic dysregulation. In persons with physical alterations to the blood vessels, such as vascular wall thickening or coronary artery plaque, otherwise normal autonomic and endocrine adjustments to exercise may cause abnormal responses. Exaggerated blood pressure rises during treadmill exercise are a sign of existing or impending hypertension (Jackson et al., 1983; Wilson, Sung, Pincomb, & Lovallo, 1990; Wilson & Meyer, 1981). Such studies suggest that preclinical alterations in vascular resistance (Lovallo & al'Absi, 1998) can cause a disproportionate rise in blood pressure relative to an otherwise normal demand for blood flow. In such cases, the abnormal reactivity may be an indicator of underlying pathology, thus serving as a marker of disease but not necessarily acting as a cause.

Though we may often look to central nervous system determinants of differences in reactivity, it is possible that in some instances persons are more reactive because of alterations in peripheral mechanisms. In this case, a person might have exaggerated responses to a stressor without any alteration in appraisals, emotions, or centrally induced alterations in endocrine or autonomic outflow. For example, persons may cluster into groups on the basis of alpha- and beta-adrenoreceptor sensitivity and hence may have different cardiovascular responses to otherwise similar degrees of central activation (Mills et al., 1994; Mills, Dimsdale, Ziegler, Berry, & Bain, 1990). Similarly, the heart rate response to a mental arithmetic challenge may be associated with peripheral adrenoreceptor function (Mills et al., 1990).

Finally, persons developing hypertension may have altered vascular reactivity that is of peripheral origin, resulting in enhanced blood pressure responses to pharmacological challenges. One such challenge is caffeine, which potentiates the action of norepinephrine at the sympathetic nerve terminal and elevates peripheral vascular resistance. In studying blood pressure responses to caffeine, we saw progressively greater pressure rises in 185 subjects stratified into four risk groups, ranging from low-risk controls to medicated hypertensives (Hartley et al., 2000). The subjects in these separate studies reported no differences in subjective activation or distress to the caffeine or to stressful tasks (Lovallo et al., 1991; Pincomb et al., 1996; Sung, Lovallo, Whitsett, & Wilson, 1995). In another study, caffeine given to borderline hypertensives induced a more prolonged increase in blood pressure over an hour of mental stress (Lovallo, al'Absi, & Pincomb, 2000), again without differences in reported activation or distress (al'Absi, Everson, & Lovallo, 1995). These studies suggest that the high-risk groups were experiencing caffeine and the stressors in the same way as the low-risk subjects. Caffeine raises blood pressure by actions at the blood vessel wall (Pincomb et al., 1996). The absence of self-report differences between the groups and the known peripheral actions of caffeine strongly suggest that the pressure differences between hypertension risk groups were peripheral in origin.

In a similar vein, Folkow (1990) argued that once structural remodeling of resistance vessels has begun and vascular wall thickening has begun to progress, blood pressure responses to any stimulus that raises pressure, whether of central or peripheral origin, will result in a disproportionate response because of the pressure flow dynamics of an increasingly restrictive vessel. In some studies, hypertensives have been shown to exhibit greater blood pressure responses to a stressor than normotensives in the absence of group differences in norepinephrine or epinephrine levels (Dimsdale, Ziegler, Mills, Delehanty, & Berry, 1990). Such evidence is again consistent with hypertensives' having a more reactive vascular system able to cause greater responses even when central influences are not altered. The lack of self-reported differences in arousal or affect in relation to the enhanced blood pressure rises in the studies reported above argues for the action of such peripheral factors, alone in the case of resting data, or driven by activity originating in higher centers during states of stress.

Health Outcomes Related to Cardiovascular and Endocrine Response Tendencies

There are suggestive data indicating that long-term exposure to stress, and presumably prolonged, frequent sympathetic activation, may lead to increased rates of disease (Lovallo & Wilson, 1992). For example, air traffic controllers working in high-workload control centers showed a higher prevalence of hypertension than those working in low-volume centers (Cobb & Rose, 1973). Presumably the long-term stress of such employment elicited greater rates of hypertension among hypertension-prone workers. In an innovative study, Italian nuns living in a cloistered convent were found to have no increase in blood pressure over 25 years. By comparison, control women from the surrounding community showed the typical age-related increase over the same time (Timio et al., 1988).

Individuals living near Three Mile Island during the nuclear accident who believed the area was contaminated with radioactivity showed elevated urinary cortisols months after the event. Other evidence indicates that traumatic stress during natural disasters can produce immediate changes in health. The second greatest cause of mortality in the 1993 Los Angeles earthquake was sudden death due to heart attack. The 1989 Loma Prieta earthquake near San Francisco produced severe dissociative reactions and longer-term psychological sequelae. Other examples of the health effects of traumatic stress were discussed in Chapter 6.

These studies of stress and health suggest that we should expect the greatest future health consequences in persons having the largest sympathetic and endocrine responses. There is evidence that this is the case, both in cardiovascular disease risk and in altered immune system function. We have noted that persons may differ in how they respond to stress because of personality traits, such as hostility, or because of hypothalamically mediated differences in reactivity tendencies. We have reason to believe that both types of individual difference in response to stress can contribute uniquely to differences in health.

Personality Mediators of Risk for Premature Mortality

There are at least two lines of evidence that personality characteristics and their associated perceptions, evaluations, and emotions may have long-term health consequences. The first line of evidence concerns the effects of hopelessness on health, described in Chapter 7. We noted that persons expressing feelings of hopelessness were at substantially increased risk of premature death due to all causes, including cardiovascular diseases over the next several years, even though these persons were normally healthy at the start of the study (Everson, Goldberg, et al., 1996; Everson et al., 1997).

The second line of evidence indicates that hostility is also a psychological contributor to negative health outcomes. Williams and colleagues found that persons high in cynical hostility as measured by the Cook-Medley (Hostility) Ho Scale were at increased risk of death due to all causes (Barefoot et al., 1983). In light of the studies by Suarez and Everson reviewed above, we may speculate that hostile persons perceive many social situations in a negative light, produce feelings of hostility, and develop exaggerated physiological responses. Such situational appraisals and their accompanying responses may be at the root of the elevated death rates seen in highly hostile persons. We at present do not have data on the physiological response tendencies of hopeless persons and therefore do not have an equally plausible hypothesis for the mechanistic links is such persons.

Cardiovascular Reactivity as a Mediator of Disease Risk

We now turn to evidence supporting the idea that exaggerated cardiovascular response tendencies may also have negative health outcomes. Although this area is too large to review in detail, there are some noteworthy points to cover.

In 1932, Hines and Brown reasoned that because hypertensives have large blood pressure responses to stress, normotensives who spontaneously show large responses may in turn be at high risk for hypertension. This early version of the reactivity hypothesis was based on the psychosomatic idea that exaggerated responses to stress were evidence of a flaw in the cardiovascular systems of highly reactive persons and that this flaw might ultimately result in essential hypertension (Alexander, 1950). Evidence has slowly accumulated suggesting that exaggerated cardiovascular reactivity in fact does predict greater risk for future cardiovascular disease.

Manuck and colleagues tested heart rate reactivity and heart disease development in monkeys living in social groups. They tested heart rate responses by approaching a group's living quarters wearing a large "monkey glove," indicating that one monkey was about to be captured for some sort of procedure. Monkeys view this as a substantial stressor, and their heart rate responses may be presumed to accompany negative emotions and evaluations of threat. Several years after being classified as to reactivity, the monkeys were sacrificed to examine their coronary arteries for atherosclerosis. The highly reactive monkeys had more extensive areas of atherosclerotic disease and greater progression of their lesions (Manuck, Kaplan, Adams, & Clarkson, 1989). This effect could be eliminated by beta-blockers, indicating that reduction of the cardiac responses or their related emotions could improve health outcomes in the highly reactive monkeys.

There is also suggestive evidence that large cardiovascular responses to stress indicate greater risk for hypertension in later years. The first line of work shows that normotensive young men at high risk for hypertension, based on family history and moderately elevated systolic blood pressures, have the largest blood pressure responses to mental arithmetic stress (al'Absi et al., 1995). These results are consistent with the reactivity hypothesis: namely, that the greater reactivity of the high-risk persons either is a marker of greater hypertension risk or contributes in a causal way.

The second line of work relates greater cardiovascular stress responses to increased rates of hypertension in later years, as originally predicted by Hines and Brown (1932). Persons with the largest blood pressure responses to cold pressor stimulation had the greatest cumulative incidence of hypertension 30 years later (Menkes et al., 1989). Also, men with the highest systolic blood pressures during a reaction-time task using electric shock as the incentive had the highest blood pressures 10 to 15 years later (Light, Dolan, Davis, & Sherwood, 1992; Light et al., 1999). Everson and colleagues showed that men having the largest blood pressure rises in anticipation of a bicycle exercise stress test had the greatest prevalence of hypertension 4 years later (Everson, Kaplan, Goldberg, & Salonen, 1996) and were more likely to suffer from cerebral stroke, a frequent complication of hypertension (Everson et al., 2001). Prospective data in a cohort of British men showed that blood pressure responses to a paced mental arithmetic task predicted blood pressure elevations over the next 5 years (Carroll, Ring, Hunt, Ford, & Macintyre, 2003). Similarly, stress blood pressure reactions in children predict adolescent blood pressures (Matthews, Salomon, Brady, & Allen, 2003). In a related vein, elevated cardiovascular reactivity to mental stressors is related to elevations in blood levels of low-density lipoprotein cholesterol, a significant risk factor for coronary heart disease (Fredrikson, Lundberg, & Tuomisto, 1991).

Immune System Alterations, Cardiovascular Reactivity, and Health

Referring to our discussion of stress mechanisms and immune function in Chapter 8, we noted that both sympathetic activity and cortisol secretion are important modulators of immune function. We should therefore expect that persons having the greatest responses to stress will have the greatest modulation of immune system function. The studies we reviewed earlier indicated that heart rate responses to mental stress are related both to greater evidence of global sympathetic activation and to greater cortisol secretion to appropriate situational cues, strengthening this contention. In fact, recent work suggests that sympathetically mediated cardiac responses to stressors such as mental arithmetic and public speaking are also related to alterations in indicators of immune system function. Cacioppo and colleagues preselected high– and low–heart rate–reactive men on the basis of reactions to a speech stressor, during which the low reactors showed a heart rate response of +5 bpm and the high reactors +30 bpm. Three weeks later, these reactivity groups were retested on a mental arithmetic challenge (Sgoutas-Emch et al., 1994). As expected, the high–heart rate reactors showed larger heart rate and blood pressure responses to the mental arithmetic tasks and had larger cortisol responses. The highly reactive subjects had the greatest increases in natural killer-cell activation, indexed by the ability of their natural killer cells to attack and kill infected cells in a laboratory assay. Note that this greater reactivity tendency was associated in this brief stressor with enhanced cortisol responses and enhanced immune function, not with depressed immune function. We suspect that this is an example of the ability of cortisol to increase immune system function in response to mild stressors of brief duration.

Indeed, other work suggests that cortisol reactivity predicts depressed immune function as indicated by reactivation of latent viral infection. Elderly women and female undergraduates worked on a combination of mental arithmetic and a speech stressor. Women with the largest cortisol responses had the greatest evidence of latent virus reactivation as indicated by their higher antibody titers to the Epstein-Barr virus (Cacioppo et al., 1995). The higher viral titers in the more reactive women are considered an indicator of recent reactivation of the virus, thus suggesting a decrease in immune system surveillance of this normally latent virus.

The overall pattern of these results shows that autonomic function, endocrine function, and immune system function are linked in states of stress. This pattern shows a significant degree of individual variation, leading us to conclude that individuals differ in centrally determined autonomic responsivity and that such differences can potentially have consequences for immune system function and presumably for long-term health. Clearly, much work remains to be done in this intriguing area.

Discussion

The emergence of an integrated field of study incorporating neurophysiology, personality theory, autonomic and endocrine function, immune system activity, and health provides us with a very powerful set of tools to take a multilevel approach to our understanding of health and disease. The information reviewed above leads us to consider that there may well be systematic relationships between the tendency of some persons to be highly reactive to stress and to also suffer more negative health consequences. We have attempted to systematize disparate lines of research using our model of centrally determined stress responses presented in Chapter 6. This allows a top-to-bottom integration of how the system could be altered by what we think and feel, and in turn these tendencies to think and feel in certain ways may have a strong biological and experiential basis.

Ultimately, our physiological behaviors accompanying our evaluations and emotions become major influences on our bodies.

We presented evidence that individual differences in stress response can arise out of differences in situational appraisals and differences in resulting emotional responses, pointing to activity in prefrontal and temporal structures. We presented other evidence that response biases can also be determined by activational differences at the hypothalamus. We then presented evidence that both psychologically and physiologically based reactivity differences could result in impaired health.

The ultimate value of attempting to integrate information on evaluative processes, emotions, and autonomic-endocrine outflow into our models of disease etiology is twofold. First, we will be able to view health and disease as the outcome of psychophysiological processes encompassing both the behavior and physiology of the individual. Second, the individual-differences approach described here helps us understand more clearly the mechanisms relating behavior to health and disease, and it provides us with ways to identify persons at greatest risk of disease.

If we return to our basic question concerning how ideas can come to have power over our bodies, we can now see that there are meaningful relationships between evaluations, mood states, and central nervous system function in relation to emotion tendencies. These in turn determine autonomic and endocrine outflow. The evidence reviewed here suggests that there are indeed systematic differences between persons in their reactions to psychological stressors. These differences translate into consistent differences in endocrine impacts on the immune system and autonomic alterations on cardiovascular structures. But our list of targets for such peripheral changes, limited to immune and cardiovascular functions, is not complete. These two classes of outcome are the best studied to date, and they fit neatly into the framework of this book. But we have no reason to believe that individual differences in psychological stress response and health consequences are limited to the influences of cardiovascular reactions and adrenocortical responses. There are likely to be other mechanistic relationships between differences in the activity of the central nervous system and health.

Summary

In this chapter, we have reviewed evidence that persons may have different ways of responding to potential threats. Persons may differ systematically in how they *perceive and evaluate* situations they face. These differences may determine consistent differences in emotional responses. For example, persons having strongly negative emotions in response to a variety of situations are likely to have greater autonomically mediated cardiovascular reactions, even ones inappropriate to the situation at hand. Persons may also differ in their *hypothalamic and brainstem* activational tendencies, even when they do not differ in their perceptions and emotional reactions. Research on persons with greater heart rate responses shows considerable stability of such responses across situations and over time, pointing to a physiological basis for this reactivity. Studies in groups at high risk for hypertension show increased cortisol reactivity in the absence of affective or evaluative differences. Finally, other studies point to *peripheral sources* of reactivity differences between groups. Whether the source of exaggerated physiological activation is an emotional response bias, such as trait hostility, an autonomic response bias, or a peripheral difference, the exaggerated reactivity has the same impact on the periphery. These individual differences in stress reactivity may predict differences in health outcomes. More generally, these differences in reactivity to mental stressors indicate that the ways in which ideas can influence the body can vary systematically from person to person and become major predictors of health and disease.

Further Reading

Light, K. C. (2001). Hypertension and the reactivity hypothesis: The next generation. *Psychosomatic Medicine, 63,* 744–746.

A commentary on refinement of contemporary reactivity hypotheses in testing relationships to disease risk.

Turner, J. R. (1994). *Cardiovascular reactivity and stress: Patterns of physiological response.* New York: Plenum.

A very thorough coverage of cardiovascular reactivity research in relation to individual differences.

Turner, J. R., Sherwood, A., & Light, K. C. (Eds.). (1992). *Individual differences in cardiovascular response to stress.* New York: Plenum.

An extended discussion of individual differences in stress reactivity, including factors not dealt with here, such as reactivity differences due to gender and race.

Treiber, F. A., Kamarck, T., Schneiderman, N., Sheffield, D., Kapuku, G., & Taylor, T. (2003). Cardiovascular reactivity and development of preclinical and clinical disease states. *Psychosomatic Medicine, 65*(1), 46–62.

A thorough review of evidence linking reactivity to health and disease, with a discussion of modifier variables and assessment of future research needs.

12

Behavior, Stress, and Health

A t the beginning of this book, we asked how ideas could come to have power over our bodies. From the point of a truly behavioral medicine, we need to understand how all of our behaviors, including our thoughts and emotions, can relate with our physical selves. As we have tried to show, the study of psychological stress is perfectly suited to this task because it forces us to consider how our perceptions and interpretations of the world can result in negative emotions and how these can change the autonomic and endocrine influences on the rest of the body.

The Historical Dilemma of Mind-Body Dualism

We have addressed the mind-body relationship and the concept of psychological stress from a historical perspective. Mind-body dualism limits how we think about ourselves, and it also limits our science of biology and medicine. Our dualistic view creates barriers to an understanding of how the apparently nonphysical thoughts that seem to occupy our heads come to have influence over our bodies. As a result, we have had a very difficult time developing a framework for medicine that incorporates behavior as both a cause and a cure.

We contrasted traditional biomedicine with an emerging theoretical framework for behavioral medicine. We argued that because of our adherence to a dualistic view of mind and body, the development of a mechanistic physiology and neurophysiology has excluded our experiential, evaluative, goal-directed existence from our biology. As a result, we lack ways to model how thoughts may affect health. This in turn has posed obstacles to the development of a behavioral medicine.

Behavioral medicine calls for removal of the metaphysical dichotomy between mind and body. It calls for us to theorize differently about the influence of perceptions, thoughts, and emotions on our biology. Ultimately, it may allow us to consider social processes and culture as causal agents in health and disease. The advantage of this behavioral agenda for medicine is that we may then develop mechanistically rigorous theories that allow for behavioral causes as well as behavioral treatments of disease and maintenance of health.

The starting point for this effort seems to lie in how psychologists conceptualize cognitive processes in relation to brain function. Traditional cognitive approaches emerged in the 1960s from an earlier doctrinaire behaviorist psychology. In the school of radical behaviorism, biology was banished as a dangerous form of reductionism. Cognitive psychology evolved as an abiological field of study, one that relied heavily on computer metaphors. Ulrich Neisser (1967) strongly adhered to this perspective, and his preeminence as a founder of cognitive psychology helped define the trend:

> First, let us consider the familiar parallel between man and computer. Although it is an inadequate analogy in many ways, it may suffice for this purpose. The task of a psychologist trying to understand human cognition is analogous to that of a man trying to discover how a computer has been programmed. In particular, if the program seems to store and reuse information, he would like to know by what "routines" or "procedures" this is done. Given this purpose, he will not care much whether his particular computer stores information in magnetic cores or in thin films; he wants to understand the program, not the "hardware." By the same token, it would not help the psychologist to know that memory is carried by RNA as opposed to some other medium. He wants to understand its utilization, not its incarnation. (p. 6)

This doctrine encourages researchers to continue to separate the mysterious software of the mind from the concrete hardware of the brain. The problem with this view is that in our computers, the software has a separate existence from the hardware. The software runs on the hardware without altering it. This computer metaphor fails to help us appreciate how the operation of our thoughts and emotions is completely at one with the neurophysiological and biochemical behavior of our brains. Other writers have addressed this problem under the rubric of establishing a neurosciences approach to the study of affective processes (Davidson & Sutton, 1995) and cognition (Albright, Kandel, & Posner, 2000).

Instead, we will argue that our thoughts are a *fundamental* expression of the behavior of our brains and that it is not possible for us to have thoughts and feelings that do not involve actions of the brain. However, this recognition has been slow in coming, and the formation of a tight linkage between neural events and behaviors has a remarkably short history in the study of behavior. For example, the first known relationship between a behavior and a definable neuronal event did not occur until 1969, when Miller (1995) reported that norepinephrine released by nerve terminals in the hypothalamus elicited eating behavior in rats. The striking advances in the modification of brain structure during development, illustrated in our review of Levine and Meaney's studies in Chapter 10, show us the power of social interactions to affect the neural structure of the brain. These changes in turn affected the behavior and ultimately the health of the animals throughout life.

Matter and Behavior

Though space limits our ability to deal with the mind-body problem in depth, we will briefly consider why it is unhelpful to view our mental activities in terms of the Cartesian Ghost in the Machine. We will also propose the form of a solution: that all matter, by nature, is continually interactive with both energy forces and other matter. By extension, it is fundamentally contradictory to devise special rules to guide the behavior of matter that is organized biologically. Putting this another way, it is incorrect to think of biological systems and the matter that composes them as different from all other forms of matter. Similarly, the physical principles that govern matter govern biological systems, however nonobvious that governance may be. Considering our human psychology, this unitary principle is not contradicted by our self-awareness or our ability to talk about ourselves in books such as this one.

As we noted in Chapter 1, Descartes imagined the body without the soul to be an inert entity otherwise identical to a clock or other machine. Some external source of energy was needed to wind the springs to make the clock move. This view was part of the generally held 17th-century attitude that all matter was fundamentally incapable of action. Adam Ferguson, writing at that time, asserted, "That matter can never put itself in motion is allowed by all men" (quoted in Toulmin, 1967, p. 823). In fact, Isaac Newton argued that matter could only react to direct pressure or contact from other matter outside itself. The same matter and energy distinction was considered true for living things. Anticipating the vitalists who antagonized Bernard in the

19th century, Giovanni Borelli argued 200 years earlier that muscles were passive organs that could move the limbs only when acted on by the "motive faculty of the soul" (Toulmin, 1967, p. 824).

The view that matter was inert was opposed only by a small minority of writers such as Mettrie (Toulmin, 1967), who argued that matter was not fundamentally unmoving but in fact *inherently* active. Like Mettrie, we wish to argue that matter is not inert but inherently active and self-interacting and that our consciousness proceeds naturally from our biology. Consciousness should therefore be seen as a result of the elementary structure of our central nervous system in relation to its higher-order organization. This approach to consciousness is consistent with current views of brain structure and its complexity in relation to the development of consciousness, self-consciousness, and consciousness of other consciousnesses (Dasser, Ulbaek, & Premack, 1989; Premack, 2004). To clarify the relationship between structure and function in the nervous system, we consider Mettrie's idea using some simpler examples.

As Toulmin (1967) pointed out, physics long ago abandoned the Newtonian idea that matter consisted of otherwise inactive particles colliding only when acted on by some outside force. This older style of physics viewed material states and energy processes as fundamentally separate things. In contrast, for the past century, matter has been seen by physics as constantly interacting with itself. More correctly, matter and energy are held to be different manifestations of an underlying unity. Using a term from psychology, we may say that matter is *fundamentally behaving*. Considering matter at its most elementary level, this view applies in describing the structure-function of quarks, the candidates for the fundamental constituents of matter. We use the term *structure-function* here because the quantum mechanical description of quarks includes both their energetic behavior and their physical properties in a single descriptive phrase, so to speak. Quarks have the properties of charge, charm, and color. Each of these properties expresses not a fixed aspect of the quark's physical makeup but consistent rules for how quarks behave in relation to their physical properties. So for quarks, their material properties and their behaviors are inseparable. The same statements hold true for more complex particles such as protons and neutrons, and for atoms and molecules, even though the rules specifying structure and behavior become extraordinarily complex even at this level.

Without further proof, we simply argue that what holds for simpler particles also holds true for more complex constructions of matter.

What about biology? If we agree that biological material is constructed of the same simpler stuff that makes up all material things, we can begin to see that the distinction between material things that are biological and material things that are not biological is already arbitrary. We can then make the same series of arguments here: namely, the structure of biological entities determines that they behave in accord with their structure and that more complex biological entities are accordingly capable of increasingly great ranges of behavior. It is not reasonable to have a complex biological structure capable of behavior that is not emergent from its structure.

We may start by considering the behavior of a simple biological entity, the sodium channel. Found on virtually all lipid membranes in the body, the sodium channel is responsible for keeping most of the sodium outside our neurons and for opening on command to allow sodium to enter in the process of initiating another action, such as calcium channel activity or a nerve firing. Figure 12.1 is a recent illustration of the sodium channel. The sodium channel starts as a specific sequence of amino acids that form themselves into a long protein molecule. With the help of chaperon proteins, these one-dimensional strings of amino acids fold up on themselves in complex ways to form three-dimensional protein molecules. Sodium channels have a unique three-dimensional shape that is a direct result of the specific sequence of amino acids in the original chain. The completed protein has new behavioral capabilities that are a direct result of its emergent three-dimensional structure. A sodium channel, when fully formed and embedded in its lipid membrane, can change shape in predictable ways given specific stimuli in its microenvironment. The channels have a central pore through which sodium ions may pass, and the pore has a series of gates that keep sodium ions out and let them in on command. It has specific external domains that respond to the environment to increase or decrease the neuron's resting potential and the strength of its discharge.

In recognition of the relationship between structure and function, neurobiologists study the behavior of the sodium channel by altering its structure in known ways and examining the resulting changes in function. Such investigation tells us how the internal gates work to regulate ion flow. It helps us to see how sodium ions are able to tumble through the pore itself. The success of this research agenda leads us to conclude that the functioning of the sodium channel is inseparable from its structure and that any change in the physical makeup of the original amino acid chain must produce a reliable change in how the molecule functions. As in the case of quarks, we may say that the behavior of the sodium channel is determined by its structure, even though the sodium channel is orders of magnitude more complex than a quark.

Because a sodium channel is far simpler than a brain, it is perhaps easier to intuitively grasp how the amino acid structure of the channel

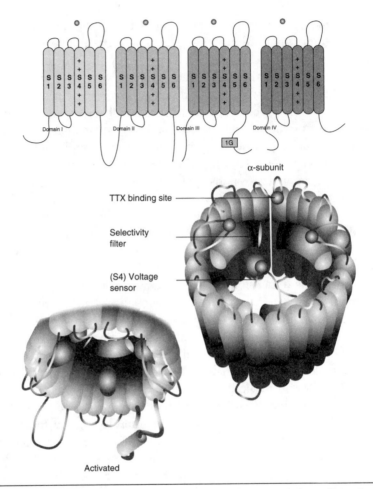

Figure 12.1   The relationship between structure and function in the sodium channel. The chain of amino acids that forms the molecule is precisely woven through the lipid membrane of the cell to form a three-dimensional structure. The resulting sodium channel has four domains that together form a central pore capable of regulating the flow of sodium ions across the membrane using a series of four molecular gates. The actions of the gates are controlled by voltage-sensitive segments of the molecule that alter the state of the gates. Redrawn from Bear, M. F., Connors, B. W., & Paradiso, M. A. (2001). *Neuroscience: Exploring the Brain* (2nd ed.). Philadelphia: Lippincott, Williams, & Wilkins. Copyright © 2002 Lippincott Williams & Wilkins. Used with permission.

determines its behavior. In the case of an entire brain, the argument may have less intuitive appeal, and there is no simple substitute to prove the case. However, we should return to our thoughts in Chapters 1 and 2 about the mind-body problem in medicine. We noted that our science is grounded on the premise that the rules describing the behavior of simple things are fundamentally the same as those for complex things. That is, the world does not acquire categorically (ontologically) new entities simply by virtue of things becoming structurally more complex. By extension, we should consider that the rules guiding structure-function relationships should hold in principle for complex combinations of neurons and for whole brains, just as they hold for the far simpler sodium channels.

This is not to underestimate the difficulties in forming useful models of neural structures and their related functions. For example, in the case of the sodium channel, science has been inquiring into the conduction of nerve impulses for more than 250 years. The study of whole brains will certainly take a long time. In spite of these empirical and conceptual difficulties, the willingness to examine behavior and biology in a unified way will continue to provide useful insights, including the effect of mental activity on the structure of the brain.

As a step in this direction, it is now possible to relate changes in brain activity to the subject's performance of specific cognitive tasks (Kosslyn & Koenig, 1995) and his or her experience of given emotional states. But can the behavior of the system also change its biology? Recent studies suggest clearly that it can. Patients undergoing 10 weeks of cognitive-behavioral therapy for obsessive-compulsive disorder were shown to have changes in limbic system activity as measured by positron emission tomography. The observed changes mimicked those produced by pharmacological treatment for the same disorder (Schwartz, Stoessel, Baxter, Martin, & Phelps, 1996). Similar behavioral effects on neural systems are seen in studies of behavioral dominance in the crayfish (Barinaga, 1996). When pairs of crayfish fight to establish dominance, the winner begins to secrete more serotonin and the loser secretes less. The serotonin primes the nervous system of the dominant crayfish to function more effectively in aggressive behaviors. We see here another example of the effect of behavior on the long-term state of the nervous system and the ultimate elicitation of new or altered behaviors. These changed behaviors will affect the nervous system in new ways, with yet further consequences for behavior. Finally, to return to contemporary studies of consciousness within evolutionary psychology, the guiding principle is that consciousness has evolved along with complexity of brain structures, in particular, with evolution of the prefrontal cortex. These examples of behavioral-structural interactions provide evidence that the principles guiding our study of emotions and behaviors need not be fundamentally different from the language we use to describe our physiological states and processes. Such evidence suggests that psychological stressors and their related emotions may well affect our brains and our bodies. In the past several years, research has produced striking examples of how stress and nurturing both act to powerfully shape the behavior and brain function of the individual, as discussed in Chapter 10.

Although this recognition is fundamental to resolving the paradox of mind and body, it does not answer the most difficult questions, such as how the organized behavior of collections of neurons ultimately becomes our subjective experience or how our sense of self-continuity over time arises from this neuronal activity. However, a number of highly creative approaches to these matters are being taken in the field of the neurosciences (Churchland, 1986; Damasio, 1994).

Behavioral Medicine in Relation to Traditional Medicine

Moving from the broad framework of the mind-body problem to the question at hand, we should be equally concerned with how a behavioral medicine could differ from traditional medicine. Our views of health, disease, and treatment will be strongly influenced by the models we use to describe these processes. In Chapter 2, we considered a series of models of disease viewed within a traditional framework of biomedicine and then described how these would differ within a conceptually broader behavioral medicine perspective. The key distinction between these two views is that in a behavioral medicine, it becomes permissible to think about how conscious processes can have causal agency in the body. This in turn allows us to think about the possibility that social and even cultural processes can affect health.

This shift from a view of the body as a passive agent, acted upon by a pathogen or a treatment, to an active entity that takes in information, evaluates it, and reacts to those evaluations not only opens up new ways of thinking about what makes us sick but also permits new ways of thinking about what can make us well (Foss & Rothenberg, 1988).

To focus these broad questions onto the narrower topic of this book, we introduced in Chapter 3 a history of the concept of stress. This historical description allowed us to see the roots of the Cartesian dilemma in our current model of biology. Notably, Claude Bernard had to contend with the antimechanistic vitalists then active in French intellectual circles. Because the vitalists argued that the body was acted on internally by a nonphysical vital force, Bernard was compelled to argue against this physiological version of the Ghost in the Machine and to assert a mechanistic epistemology for the science of physiology. This effort successfully established the basis for considering lawful physical relationships in traditional physiology, but it did not readily give us a way to think about how psychological events could alter brain and bodily function. So, ironically, the Cartesian dualism persisted in our thinking about the workings of the mind even after the mysterious vital forces had been banished from the working of the rest of the body. Partly for this reason, modern medicine has not incorporated behavior into its conceptual framework.

Our consideration of physical and psychological stress gives us one way to think about the relationship between psychological events and physiological events in the body. We have proposed in this book that laying down a mechanistic model of physical stress leads more naturally to an understanding of how psychological events can also come to act as stressors.

Systems Organization and Stress

In Chapter 4, we described the normal modes of bodily regulation in order to consider the disruptions caused by psychological stress. We noted that homeostatic regulation involved layers of control over each organ and tissue, starting with the local regulation designed into each of these and proceeding to increasingly elaborate levels of nervous system and hormonal regulation, up to and including the functions of the hypothalamus. Higher levels in the system therefore modulate and coordinate the activity of lower levels.

We then discussed in Chapter 5 the admittedly arbitrary distinction between physiological and psychological stressors. We noted that in both cases common output pathways and peripheral mechanisms were engaged. The essential difference is that in physiological stress, exemplified by exercise stress, the major sources of perturbation to the system are the metabolic demands on fuel homeostasis and feedback from working muscles, with the added influence of mental effort. In the case of psychological stressors, the major sources of perturbation are descending influences originating in higher brain centers and operating without regard to physiological demands (Turner & Carroll, 1985).

Chapters 6 and 7 are the focal point of this book. We described how the central nervous system is equipped to carry out a continuous monitoring of the environment and prepares constantly to make adaptive responses. This process is associated with a continual flow of emotional experience and motivational states resulting in physiological outputs. Psychologically, the generation of emotions may occur to present threats or to imagined, remembered, and anticipated threats. The frontal cortex appears to provide an essential structural basis for the operation of working memory. Working memory is able to produce a realistic representation of events, including those that are not actually present. The prefrontal cortex, in its relationship to the limbic system, was therefore shown to operate on processes typically considered purely psychological in nature—ideas, perceptions, and memories. In response to these imagined or recalled events, we produce the same stream of emotions and their related autonomic and endocrine outputs that originally evolved to deal with immediate physical threats. This model provides us with one answer to our basic question of how ideas could come to have power over our bodies.

The layered organization of the system, with local metabolic controls at the bottom and ganglionic and spinal reflexes, brainstem reflexes, hypothalamic regulation, and ultimately cortical and limbic controls at the top, allows us to think about how cortical activity associated with evaluations and emotions can alter the functioning of the lower levels. Using this conception, we may properly argue that the prefrontal cortex applies the highest level of control to the regulation of bodily processes. In the context of a model of psychological stress, we can therefore think about how mental states can produce fight-or-flight responses in the body.

We also noted in Chapter 5 that the distinction between physical and psychological stress was really arbitrary because in a conscious person all physical stressors have a psychological component. For this reason, there may be no such thing as a pure physical stressor, although there may be pure psychological stressors.

Psychological Stress and Its Consequences

With the model described in Chapters 6 and 7, we were able to talk meaningfully about the consequences of psychological stress. In Chapter 8, we showed how psychological processes and immune system function are linked. Most interestingly, we were able to draw from a variety of creative studies that have capitalized on naturally occurring stressors to measure changes in immune system functions in persons' daily lives. Such work is relevant to the human condition, and it gives us an increasingly clear view of the impact of psychological events on health. This work tends to be correlational, matching up immune system changes with experience of lack of control or ceaseless struggle in daily life. What remains is to understand how the causal chain of events operates from the experience of life to altered emotions, limbic system function, and altered hypothalamic and autonomic function. Most importantly, we need to know much more about how practical, minimally invasive measures of immune system function can be used to reflect actual disease susceptibility.

In Chapter 9, we dealt with the severe, even disastrous effects that feelings of complete helplessness can engender in humans and laboratory animals. We discussed examples from anthropological observation of persons dying as an apparent result of witchcraft, but closer to our own experience we gave examples of death due to the psychological experience of fear and helplessness in the face of wars and natural disasters. Although these are dramatic demonstrations of psychological effects on health, they are far removed from everyday experience and are extreme relative to more chronic psychological stress experienced on a daily basis.

We then turned to a series of animal studies on the influences of coping and control over aversive events. These provide an excellent basis for understanding some key physiological causes of the body's response to psychological stress. They illustrate graphically that removal of adequate coping options during exposure to aversive stimulation can result in severe physical consequences in the form of ulcers and other tissue pathology. Most interestingly, these effects are paralleled by changes in central nervous system noradrenergic and serotonergic transmitter systems. These changes in turn produce behavioral manifestations of mood disorders such as depression. Returning to the Lazarus model of psychological stress, we note that coping and control in the face of aversive threats are the major determinants of psychologically induced stress responses. Similarly, reducing the experience of helplessness can powerfully avert the psychophysiological consequences of the physical stressor. These outcomes of stress exposure increase or decrease as a consequence of the shaping of the animal's psychological set: Helplessness worsens outcomes, positive feedback about safety improves them.

Chapter 10 is entirely new for this second edition. In it we summarize emerging themes from work that has been in progress for some time, namely the studies of early nurturing and stress in rat models. The recent reports by Michael Meaney and his group allow increasingly definitive statements about the nature of these early experiences in regulating gene expression over the life span of the individual animal. In the case of the nurturing model, this happens to result in differences in central serotonin activity and expression of genes for glucocorticoid receptors. The result is that the animal has a greatly altered behavioral relationship to its environment, being more exploratory and less anxious. Females so nurtured become nurturant mothers themselves. We also discussed the groundbreaking work of Caspi and colleagues, who have provided the best existing evidence on the interaction between a genetic vulnerability and the effects of life experience. The events experienced by the members of the New Zealand cohort, particularly stressful ones, are seen to affect the health and behavior of the person in adulthood. The ability of the investigators to tie these outcomes to stress in relation to gene variations is especially impressive. These findings are important because they take the gene-environment topic out of the laboratory and into the arena of real life. For our present topic, the work on animals and humans discussed in Chapter 10 is the clearest evidence I have seen showing that what we are, and how we behave, is a result of the genetic endowment of the person as modified by the experiences the person encounters in early life as that genomic background unfolds. It would be harder to imagine a better example of the arbitrary nature of a distinction between genome and phenotype.

In Chapter 11, we showed how individual differences in psychological processes, such as hostile interpretations of social interactions, and the resulting emotions can increase the size of cardiovascular reactions to those interactions. In considering the relationships between behavioral dispositions, external circumstances, stress, and health, one is always impressed by the differences persons display in how they cope with and react to life's challenges. Ultimately a complete model of psychological stress and health will have much to say about how these individual differences arise and how they determine the nature of the person's interactions with the environment. In addition to telling us much about stress and disease, they promise to tell us even more about how persons may be highly flexible in absorbing life's challenges and avoiding their worst consequences.

Stress and Behavioral Medicine

The lessons about the negative effects of stress on health are potentially useful in helping us understand restorative processes and think about how mental activity may exert beneficial physical effects. Returning for a moment to our earlier example about the effects of psychotherapy on brain function, we presume that the altered brain activity would be accompanied by altered influences of the brain on the rest of the body.

In considering the effects of psychological stress and possible health consequences, we tend to focus on the effects of autonomic outflow and endocrine secretions on our peripheral organs. Similarly, we think of stress as affecting the operation of the immune system and reducing resistance to infectious disease. These are certainly important ways in which stress mechanisms interact with organ regulation to alter homeostasis. However, as we learn more about the brain mechanisms integrating the psychological stress response, we realize that psychological stress is likely to have important consequences for brain function. Again, the Meaney and Caspi studies are paramount examples of the interplay between behavior and brain structure and function.

The model in Chapters 6 and 7 illustrates that psychological stress is a result of activity arising in the prefrontal and limbic regions and altering the functioning of the hypothalamus and brainstem autonomic control centers. The system appears to be functionally integrated by the system of corticotropin releasing factor neurons and to involve altered activation and dysphoric moods associated with the noradrenergic fiber system and the serotonergic system. The studies of uncontrollable stress in rats indicate that altered central nervous system function is a prominent consequence of severe psychological stress. We speculated in Chapter 7 that long-lasting changes in the response tendencies of the central nervous system areas integrating the psychological stress response may be responsible for the long-term changes associated with posttraumatic stress disorder. Such changes would involve altered activation to novel or unexpected stimuli, mood alterations, and powerful autonomic and endocrine responses. In turn, this suggests that some of the most important effects of severe psychological stress are long-term alterations in the function of the brain. The hopeful message from the Meaney and Caspi studies is that nurturing and protection from severe and uncontrollable stress in early childhood can avert these consequences.

Stress Reduction and Improved Health

Because this is a book on stress, we have paid a great deal of attention to how events that we encounter can produce reactions that are negative in the sense that they can impair health. But because this book is part of a series on behavioral medicine, it seems appropriate to think about positive possibilities. If psychological events can produce stress effects in the body, it should be in principle possible for psychological events to have beneficial effects. We have paid far too little attention to the possibilities of such salubrious influences. Although many persons are prepared to think of psychological stress as impairing health, we are less well prepared to think about positive states of mind having beneficial physical effects.

We will simply argue that the more we know about the relationship between our behaviors, including our thoughts and emotions, the more likely we are to see how mental activities can act to buffer the effects of stress and increase our resistance to its negative physical effects. Turning once again to Michael Meaney's studies, nurturing in early life was seen to change gene expression and behavior in ways that we are tempted to say are beneficial, at least in a safe environment. The ability of these effects to be manifested in maternal treatment of the next generation is more far-reaching in consideration of the potential human parallels. The Caspi studies, if one inspects their published data (see Figures 10.2 and 10.4), tell us not only that harsh treatment has undesirable outcomes in vulnerable individuals but also that a benign upbringing can be protective in a vulnerable person. They also show us that some persons are hardy and resistant to the depredations of a harsh early life and to the beneficence of a nurturing one.

Summary

This chapter has been a short review of the major themes of this book. Our primary question is how ideas can come to have power over our bodies. We have used the topic of psychological stress to show that events beginning as our thoughts and perceptions of the world, and our evaluations of their meaning for ourselves, can come to have both immediate physical consequences and potential long-term health consequences. We have focused on stress in behavioral medicine and on the relationship of behavioral medicine to the larger fields of traditional medicine and biology. To lay the groundwork for understanding the relationship between behavior and health, we have argued that it is necessary to stop categorizing behavior, especially psychological or mental processes, as fundamentally different from our material makeup. This artificial distinction, in the form of the mind-body problem, makes it conceptually impossible to properly consider how behavior relates to our physical health.

We have attempted to give a more narrowly focused neurophysiological model of that process in Chapters 6 and 7 and to give examples of the workings of that process in Chapters 8–11. We hope, therefore, that by increasing our understanding of the relationships between psychological events and bodily stress responses, we will gain a greater appreciation for the relationship between behavior and health. This in turn contributes to our development of a behavioral medicine. In the largest sense, it contributes to a reframed understanding of our nature as living beings whose behavior is not separate from our physical makeup and whose health is not separate from our thoughts and emotions.

Further Reading

Churchland, P. S. (1986). *Neurophilosophy: Toward a unified science of the mind/brain.* Cambridge, MA: MIT Press.

Provides an extended discussion of the issue of mind-body relationships and the need for a dialogue among the neurosciences, psychology, and philosophy to reconceptualize ourselves in a manner that does away with the Cartesian paradox.

Damasio, A. R. (1994). *Descartes' error: Emotion, reason, and the human brain.* New York: G. P. Putnam's Sons.

A briefer account of the relationship between the mind and the brain in a thoughtfully written last chapter.

Foss, L., & Rothenberg, K. (1988). *The second medical revolution.* Boston: Shambhala.

Provides the beginnings of a biobehavioral reformulation of medicine.

Premack, D., & Premack, A. (2003). *Original intelligence: Unlocking the mystery of who we are.* New York: McGraw-Hill.

A readable account of contemporary approaches to the study of the evolution of consciousness.

References

Abercrombie, H. C., Kalin, N. H., Thurow, M. E., Rosenkranz, M. A., & Davidson, R. J. (2003). Cortisol variation in humans affects memory for emotionally laden and neutral information. *Behavioral Neuroscience, 117*, 505–516.

Ader, R., & Cohen, N. (1993). Psychoneuroimmunology: Conditioning and stress. *Annual Review of Psychology, 44*, 53–85.

al'Absi, M., Bongard, S., Buchanan, T., Pincomb, G. A., Licinio, J., & Lovallo, W. R. (1997). Cardiovascular and neuroendocrine adjustment to public speaking and mental arithmetic stressors. *Psychophysiology, 34*, 266–275.

al'Absi, M., Everson, S. A., & Lovallo, W. R. (1995). Hypertension risk factors and cardiovascular reactivity to mental stress in young men. *International Journal of Psychophysiology, 20*, 155–160.

al'Absi, M., Hugdahl, K., & Lovallo, W. R. (2002). Adrenocortical stress responses and altered working memory performance. *Psychophysiology, 39*, 95–99.

al'Absi, M., Lovallo, W. R., McKey, B. S., & Pincomb, G. A. (1994). Borderline hypertensives produce exaggerated adrenocortical responses to sustained mental stress. *Psychosomatic Medicine, 56*, 245–250.

Albright, T. D., Kandel, E. R., & Posner, M. I. (2000). Cognitive neuroscience. *Current Opinion in Neurobiology, 10*, 612–624.

Alexander, F. (1950). *Psychosomatic medicine: Its principles and applications.* New York: Norton.

Allen, M. T., Obrist, P. A., Sherwood, A., & Crowell, M. D. (1987). Evaluation of myocardial and peripheral vascular responses during reaction time, mental arithmetic and cold pressor. *Psychophysiology, 24*, 648–656.

American Heart Association. (2003). *Statistics on coronary angiography.* Retrieved November 16, 2003, from www.americanheart.org/.

Anderson, D. E., & Tosheff, J. G. (1973). Cardiac output and total peripheral resistance changes during pre-avoidance periods in the dog. *Journal of Applied Physiology, 35*, 650–654.

Antoni, M. H. (2003). Stress management effects on psychological, endocrinological, and immune functioning in men with HIV infection: Empirical support for a psychoneuroimmunological model. *Stress, 6*, 173–188.

Aston-Jones, G., Ennis, M., Pieribone, R. A., Nickell, W. T., & Shipley, M. T. (1986). The brain nucleus locus ceruleus: Restricted afferent control of a broad efferent network. *Science, 234,* 734–737.

Bachen, E. A., Manuck, S. B., Cohen, S., Muldoon, M. F., Raible, R., Herbert, T. B., et al. (1995). Adrenergic blockade ameliorates cellular immune responses to mental stress in humans. *Psychosomatic Medicine, 57,* 366–372.

Bard, P. (1928). A diencephalic mechanism for the expression of rage with special reference to the sympathetic nervous system. *American Journal of Physiology, 84,* 490–515.

Barefoot, J. C., Dahlstrom, W. G., & Williams, R. B. (1983). Hostility, CHD incidence, and total mortality: A 25-year follow-up study of 255 physicians. *Psychosomatic Medicine, 45,* 59–63.

Barinaga, M. (1996). Social status sculpts activity of crayfish neurons. *Science, 271,* 290–291.

Barker, D. J. (1990). The fetal and infant origins of adult disease. *British Medical Journal, 301,* 1111.

Baum, A. (1990). Stress, intrusive imagery, and chronic distress. *Health Psychology, 9,* 653–675.

Benson, H., & McCallie, D. P., Jr. (1979). Angina pectoris and the placebo effect. *New England Journal of Medicine, 300,* 1424–1429.

Berk, L. S., Tan, S. A., Fry, W. F., Napier, B. J., Lee, J. W., Hubbard, R. W., et al. (1989). Neuroendocrine and stress hormone changes during mirthful laughter. *American Journal of the Medical Sciences, 298,* 390–396.

Bernard, C. (1961). *An introduction to the study of experimental medicine* (H. C. Greene, Trans.). New York: Collier. (Original work published 1865)

Berntson, G. G., Cacioppo, J. T., & Quigley, K. S. (1993). Respiratory sinus arrhythmia: Autonomic origins, physiological mechanisms, and psychophysiological implications. *Psychophysiology, 30,* 183–196.

Berntson, G. G., Cacioppo, J. T., & Quigley, K. S. (1994). Autonomic cardiac control. I. Estimation and validation from pharmacological blockades. *Psychophysiology, 31,* 572–585.

Blum, K., Cull, H. G., Braverman, E. R., & Comings, D. E. (1996). Reward deficiency syndrome. *American Scientist, 84,* 132–145.

Blumenthal, J. A., Babyak, M., Wei, J., O'Connor, C., Waugh, R., Eisenstein, E., et al. (2002). Usefulness of psychosocial treatment of mental stress-induced myocardial ischemia in men. *American Journal of Cardiology, 89,* 164–168.

Blumenthal, J. A., Jiang, W., Waugh, R. A., Frid, D. J., Morris, J. J., Coleman, R. E., et al. (1995). Mental stress-induced ischemia in the laboratory and ambulatory ischemia during daily life: Association and hemodynamic features. *Circulation, 92,* 2102–2108.

Bonneau, R. H. (1994). Experimental approaches to identify mechanisms of stress-induced modulation of immunity to herpes simplex virus infection. In R. Glaser & J. K. Kiecolt-Glaser (Eds.), *Handbook of human stress and immunity* (pp. 125–160). San Diego: Academic Press.

Boone, J. L., & Anthony, J. P. (2003). Evaluating the impact of stress on systemic disease: The MOST protocol in primary care. *Journal of the American Osteopathic Association, 103,* 239–246.

Booth-Kewley, S., & Friedman, H. (1987). Psychological predictors of heart disease: A quantitative review. *Psychological Bulletin, 101,* 343–362.

Brady, J. V., Porter, R. W., Conrad, D. G., & Mason, J. W. (1958). Avoidance behavior and the development of gastroduodenal ulcers. *Journal of the Experimental Analysis of Behavior, 1,* 69–72.

Bremner, J. D., Randall, P., Scott, T. M., Bronen, R. A., Seibyl, J. P., Southwick, S. M., et al. (1995). MRI-based measurement of hippocampal volume in patients with combat-related posttraumatic stress disorder. *American Journal of Psychiatry, 152,* 973–981.

Brod, J. (1963). Hemodynamic basis of acute pressor reactions and hypertension. *British Heart Journal, 25,* 227–245.

Brown, G. L., Goodwin, F. K., Ballenger, J. C., Goyer, P. F., & Major, L. F. (1986). Aggression in humans correlates with cerebrospinal fluid amine metabolites. *Annals of the New York Academy of Sciences, 487,* 176–188.

Buchanan, T. W., & Lovallo, W. R. (2001). Enhanced memory for emotional material following stress-level cortisol treatment in humans. *Psychoneuroendocrinology, 26,* 307–317.

Buijs, R. M., van Eden, C. G., Goncharuk, V. D., & Kalsbeek, A. (2003). The biological clock tunes the organs of the body: Timing by hormones and the autonomic nervous system. *Journal of Endocrinology, 177,* 17–26.

Burns, J. F. (1988, December 4). Navy criticized on jet downing. *New York Times,* pp. 1–2.

Burns, V. E., Ring, C., Drayson, M., & Carroll, D. (2002). Cortisol and cardiovascular reactions to mental stress and antibody status following hepatitis B vaccination: A preliminary study. *Psychophysiology, 39,* 361–368.

Buss, K. A., Schumacher, J. R., Dolski, I., Kalin, N. H., Goldsmith, H. H., & Davidson, R. J. (2003). Right frontal brain activity, cortisol, and withdrawal behavior in 6-month-old infants. *Behavioral Neuroscience, 117,* 11–20.

Butterfield, F. (2002, August 21). Father steals best: Crime in an American family. *New York Times,* p. A1.

Cacioppo, J. T., & Berntson, G. G. (1994). Relationship between attitudes and evaluative space: A critical review, with emphasis on the separability of positive and negative substrates. *Psychological Bulletin, 115,* 401–423.

Cacioppo, J. T., Berntson, G. G., Binkley, P. F., Quigley, K. S., Uchino, B. N., & Fieldstone, A. (1994). Autonomic cardiac control. II. Noninvasive indices and basal response as revealed by autonomic blockades. *Psychophysiology, 31,* 586–598.

Cacioppo, J. T., Kiecolt-Glaser, J. K., Malarkey, W. B., Laskowski, B. F., Rozlog, L. A., Poehlmann, K. M., et al. (2002). Autonomic and glucocorticoid associations with the steady-state expression of latent Epstein-Barr virus. *Hormones and Behavior, 42,* 32–41.

Cacioppo, J. T., Malarkey, W. B., Kiecolt-Glaser, J. K., Uchino, B. N., Sgoutas-Emch, S. A., Sheridan, J. F., et al. (1995). Heterogeneity in neuroendocrine and immune responses to brief psychological stressors as a function of autonomic cardiac activation. *Psychosomatic Medicine, 57,* 154–164.

Cannon, W. B. (1928). The mechanism of emotional disturbance of bodily functions. *New England Journal of Medicine, 198,* 165–172.

Cannon, W. B. (1929). *Bodily changes in pain, hunger, fear, and rage* (2nd ed.). New York: Appleton.

Cannon, W. B. (1935). Stresses and strains of homeostasis (Mary Scott Newbold Lecture). *American Journal of Medical Sciences, 189,* 1–14.

Cannon, W. B. (1957). "Voodoo" death. *Psychosomatic Medicine, 19,* 182–190.

Carobrez, S. G., Gasparotto, O. C., Buwalda, B., & Bohus, B. (2002). Long-term consequences of social stress on corticosterone and IL-1beta levels in endotoxin-challenged rats. *Physiology and Behavior, 76,* 99–105.

Carroll, D., Ebrahim, S., Tilling, K., Macleod, J., & Smith, G. D. (2002). Admissions for myocardial infarction and World Cup football: Database survey. *British Medical Journal, 325,* 1439–1442.

Carroll, D., Ring, C., Hunt, K., Ford, G., & Macintyre, S. (2003). Blood pressure reactions to stress and the prediction of future blood pressure: Effects of sex, age, and socioeconomic position. *Psychosomatic Medicine, 65,* 1058–1064.

Caspi, A., McClay, J., Moffitt, T. E., Mill, J., Martin, J., Craig, I. W., et al. (2002). Role of genotype in the cycle of violence in maltreated children. *Science, 297,* 851–854.

Caspi, A., Sugden, K., Moffitt, T. E., Taylor, A., Craig, I. W., Harrington, H., et al. (2003). Influence of life stress on depression: Moderation by a polymorphism in the 5-HTT gene. *Science, 301,* 386–389.

Charvat, J., Dell, P., & Folkow, B. (1964). Mental factors and cardiovascular diseases. *Cardiologia, 44,* 124–141.

Christenfeld, N., Glynn, L. M., Phillips, D. P., & Shrira, I. (1999). Exposure to New York City as a risk factor for heart attack mortality. *Psychosomatic Medicine, 61,* 740–43.

Churchland, P. S. (1986). *Toward a unified science of the mind/brain.* Cambridge, MA: MIT Press.

Cobb, S., & Rose, R. M. (1973). Hypertension, peptic ulcer, and diabetes in air traffic controllers. *Journal of the American Medical Association, 224,* 489–492.

Cohen, S. (1994). Psychosocial influences on immunity and infectious disease in humans. In R. Glaser & J. K. Kiecolt-Glaser (Eds.), *Handbook of human stress and immunity* (pp. 301–319). San Diego: Academic Press.

Cohen, S., Hamrick, N., Rodriguez, M. S., Feldman, P. J., Rabin, B. S., & Manuck, S. B. (2002). Reactivity and vulnerability to stress-associated risk for upper respiratory illness. *Psychosomatic Medicine, 64,* 302–310.

Comings, D. E., & Blum, K. (2000). Reward deficiency syndrome: Genetic aspects of behavioral disorders. *Progress in Brain Research, 126,* 325–341.

Courtney, S. M., Petit, L., Maisog, J. M., Ungerleider, L. G., & Haxby, J. V. (1998). An area specialized for spatial working memory in human frontal cortex. *Science, 279,* 1347–1351.

Dallman, M. F. (1993). Adaptation of the hypothalamic-pituitary-adrenal axis to chronic stress. *Trends in Endocrinology and Metabolism, 4,* 62–69.

Dallman, M. F., Pecoraro, N., Akana, S. F., La Fleur, S. E., Gomez, F., Houshyar, H., et al. (2003). Chronic stress and obesity: A new view of "comfort food." *Proceedings of the National Academy of Sciences USA, 100,* 11696–11701.

Damasio, A. R. (1994). *Descartes' error: Emotion, reason, and the human brain.* New York: G. P. Putnam's Sons.

Damasio, H., Grabowski, T., Frank, R., Galaburda, A. M., & Damasio, A. R. (1994). The return of Phineas Gage: Clues about the brain from the skull of a famous patient. *Science, 264,* 1102–1105.

Dasser, V., Ulbaek, I., & Premack, D. (1989). The perception of intention. *Science, 243,* 365–367.

Davidson, R. J. (2003). Affective neuroscience and psychophysiology: Toward a synthesis. *Psychophysiology, 40,* 655–665.

Davidson, R. J., Kabat-Zinn, J., Schumacher, J., Rosenkranz, M., Muller, D., Santorelli, S. F., et al. (2003). Alterations in brain and immune function produced by mindfulness meditation. *Psychosomatic Medicine, 65,* 564–570.

Davidson, R. J., & Sutton, S. K. (1995). Affective neuroscience: The emergence of a discipline. *Current Opinion in Neurobiology, 5,* 217–224.

Davis, M. (2000). The role of the amygdala in conditioned and unconditioned fear and anxiety. In J. P. Aggleton (Ed.), *The amygdala: A functional analysis* (pp. 213–287). Oxford, UK: Oxford University Press.

Davis, M., & Whalen, P. J. (2001). The amygdala: Vigilance and emotion. *Molecular Psychiatry, 6,* 13–34.

de Vreede-Swagemakers, J. J., Gorgels, A. P., Weijenberg, M. P., Dubois-Arbouw, W. I., Golombeck, B., van Ree, J. W., et al. (1999). Risk indicators for out-of-hospital cardiac arrest in patients with coronary artery disease. *Journal of Clinical Epidemiology, 52,* 601–607.

DeBold, C., Orth, D. N., DeCherney, G. S., Jackson, R. V., Sheldon, W. R., Jr., Nicholson, W. E., et al. (1987). Corticotropin-releasing hormone: Stimulation of ACTH secretion in normal man. *Hormone and Metabolism Research, 16*(Suppl.), 8–16.

DeBold, C. R., Sheldon, W. R., DeCherney, G. S., Jackson, R. V., Alexander, A. N., Vale, W., et al. (1984). Arginine vasopressin potentiates adrenocorticotropin release induced by ovine corticotropin-releasing factor. *Journal of Clinical Investigation, 73,* 533–538.

Dembroski, T. M., MacDougall, J. M., Costa, P. T., Jr., & Grandits, G. A. (1989). Components of hostility as predictors of sudden death and myocardial infarction in the Multiple Risk Factor Intervention Trial. *Psychosomatic Medicine, 51,* 514–522.

Dent, G. W., Smith, M. A., & Levine, S. (2001). Stress-induced alterations in locus coeruleus gene expression during ontogeny. *Brain Research: Developmental Brain Research, 127,* 23–30.

Descartes, R. (1956). *Discourse on method* (L. J. Lafleur, Trans.). New York: Liberal Arts Press. (Original work published 1637)

Dieter, J. N., Field, T., Hernandez-Reif, M., Emory, E. K., & Redzepi, M. (2003). Stable preterm infants gain more weight and sleep less after five days of massage therapy. *Journal of Pediatric Psychology, 28,* 403–411.

Dimsdale, J. E., Ziegler, M., Mills, P., Delehanty, S. G., & Berry, C. (1990). Effects of salt, race, and hypertension on reactivity to stressors. *Hypertension, 16,* 573–580.

Dorn, L. D., Burgess, E. S., Friedman, T. C., Dubbert, B., Gold, P. W., & Chrousos, G. P. (1997). The longitudinal course of psychopathology in Cushing's syndrome after correction of hypercortisolism. *Journal of Clinical Endocrinology and Metabolism, 82,* 912–919.

Elstein, A. S., & Bordage, G. (1979). Psychology of clinical reasoning. In G. C. Stone, F. Cohen, & N. E. Adler (Eds.), *Health psychology: A handbook* (pp. 333–367). San Francisco: Jossey-Bass.

Engbretson, T. O., & Stoney, C. M. (1993). Cynical hostility and anger expression: Relationships to plasma lipid concentrations. *Psychosomatic Medicine, 55,* 121–122.

Engel, G. L. (1971). Sudden and rapid death during psychological stress. *Annals of Internal Medicine, 74,* 771–782.

Everson, S. A., Goldberg, D. E., Kaplan, G. A., Cohen, R. D., Pukkala, E., Tuomilehto, J., et al. (1996). Hopelessness and risk of mortality and incidence of myocardial infarction and cancer. *Psychosomatic Medicine, 58,* 113–121.

Everson, S. A., Kaplan, G. A., Goldberg, D. E., & Salonen, J. T. (1996). Anticipatory blood pressure response to exercise predicts future high blood pressure in middle-aged men. *Hypertension, 27,* 1059–1064.

Everson, S. A., Kaplan, G. A., Goldberg, D. E., & Salonen, J. T. (2000). Hypertension incidence is predicted by high levels of hopelessness in Finnish men. *Hypertension, 35,* 561–567.

Everson, S. A., Kaplan, G. A., Goldberg, D. E., Salonen, R., & Salonen, J. T. (1997). Hopelessness and 4-year progression of carotid atherosclerosis: The Kuopio Ischemic Heart Disease Risk Factor Study. *Arteriosclerosis, Thrombosis, and Vascular Biology, 17,* 1490–1495.

Everson, S. A., Lynch, J. W., Kaplan, G. A., Lakka, T. A., Sivenius, J., & Salonen, J. T. (2001). Stress-induced blood pressure reactivity and incident stroke in middle-aged men. *Stroke, 32,* 1263–1270.

Everson, S. A., McKey, B. S., & Lovallo, W. R. (1995). Effect of trait hostility on cardiovascular responses to harassment in young men. *International Journal of Behavioral Medicine, 2,* 172–191.

Felten, D. L., Cohen, N., Ader, R., Felten, S. Y., Carlson, S. L., & Roszman, T. L. (1991). Central-neural circuits involved in neural-immune interactions. In R. Ader, D. Felten, & N. Cohen (Eds.), *Psychoneuroimmunology* (2nd ed., pp. 3–25). San Diego: Academic Press.

Felten, S. Y., & Felten, D. L. (1991). Innervation of lymphoid tissue. In R. Ader, D. L. Felten, & N. Cohen (Eds.), *Psychoneuroimmunology* (2nd ed., pp. 27–69). San Diego: Academic Press.

Folkman, S. (1984). Personal control and stress and coping processes: A theoretical analysis. *Journal of Personality and Social Psychology, 46,* 839–852.

Folkow, B. (1990). "Structural factor" in primary and secondary hypertension. *Hypertension, 16,* 89–101.

Folkow, B. (1993). Physiological organization of neurohormonal responses to psychosocial stimuli: Implications for health and disease. *Annals of Behavioral Medicine, 15,* 236–244.

Foss, L., & Rothenberg, K. (1988). *The second medical revolution.* Boston: Shambhala.

Fredrikson, M., Lundberg, U., & Tuomisto, M. (1991). Serum lipid levels and cardiovascular reactivity. *Journal of Psychophysiology, 5,* 89–95.

Friedman, M., Thoresen, C. E., Gill, J. J., Ulmer, D., Powell, L. H., Price, V. A., et al. (1986). Alteration of Type A behavior and its effect on cardiac recurrences in post myocardial infarction patients: Summary results of the Recurrent Coronary Prevention Project. *American Heart Journal, 112,* 653–665.

Gilbertson, M. W., Shenton, M. E., Ciszewski, A., Kasai, K., Lasko, N. B., Orr, S. P., et al. (2002). Smaller hippocampal volume predicts pathologic vulnerability to psychological trauma. *Nature Neuroscience, 5,* 1242–1247.

Glaser, R., Kiecolt-Glaser, J. K., Bonneau, R., Malarkey, W., & Hughes, J. (1992). Stress-induced modulation of the immune response to recombinant hepatitis B vaccine. *Psychosomatic Medicine, 54,* 22–29.

Glaser, R., Kiecolt-Glaser, J. K., Speicher, C. E., & Holliday, J. E. (1985). Stress, loneliness, and changes in herpesvirus latency. *Journal of Behavioral Medicine, 8,* 249–260.

Glaser, R., Kutz, L. A., MacCallum, R. C., & Malarkey, W. B. (1995). Hormonal modulation of Epstein-Barr virus replication. *Neuroendocrinology, 62,* 356–361.

Glaser, R., Rice, J., Sheridan, J., Fertel, R., Stout, J., Speicher, C., et al. (1987). Stress-related immune suppression: Health implications. *Brain, Behavior, and Immunity, 1,* 7–20.

Glynn, L. M., Christenfeld, N., & Gerin, W. (2002). The role of rumination in recovery from reactivity: Cardiovascular consequences of emotional states. *Psychosomatic Medicine, 64,* 714–726.

Goldman-Rakic, P. S. (1996). The prefrontal landscape: Implications of functional architecture for understanding human mentation and the central executive. *Philosophical Transactions of the Royal Society of London, B: Biological Sciences, 351,* 1445–1453.

Goncharuk, V. D., Van Heerikhuize, J., Swaab, D. F., & Buijs, R. M. (2002). Paraventricular nucleus of the human hypothalamus in primary hypertension: Activation of corticotropin-releasing hormone neurons. *Journal of Comparative Neurology, 443,* 321–331.

Gray, J. A. (1987). *The psychology of fear and stress* (2nd ed.). New York: Cambridge University Press.

Gray, J. A. (1991). Neural systems, emotion and personality. In J. Maden (Ed.), *Neurobiology of learning, emotion and affect* (pp. 273–306). New York: Raven.

Greenwood-Van Meerveld, B., Gibson, M., Gunter, W., Shepard, J., Foreman, R., & Myers, D. (2001). Stereotaxic delivery of corticosterone to the amygdala modulates colonic sensitivity in rats. *Brain Research, 893,* 135–142.

Guyton, A. C., & Hall, J. E. (2000). *Textbook of medical physiology* (10th ed.). New York: W. B. Saunders.

Halloran, R. (1988, July 4). Action is defended. *New York Times,* pp. 1–2.

Harlow, J. M. (1868). Recovery from the passage of an iron bar through the head. *Journal of the Massachusetts Medical Society, 2,* 327–347.

Harrington, A. (Ed.). (1997). *The placebo effect: An interdisciplinary exploration.* Cambridge, MA: Harvard University Press.

Hartley, T. R., Sung, B. H., Pincomb, G. A., Whitsett, T. L., Wilson, M. F., & Lovallo, W. R. (2000). Hypertension risk status and effect of caffeine on blood pressure. *Hypertension, 36,* 137–141.

Hedman, A., Hjemdahl, P., Nordlander, R., & Åström, H. (1990). Effects of mental and physical stress on central haemodynamics and cardiac sympathetic nerve activity during QT interval-sensing rate-responsive and fixed rate ventricular inhibited pacing. *European Heart Journal, 11,* 903–915.

Herbert, J., Moore, G. F., de la Riva, C., & Watts, F. N. (1986). Endocrine responses and examination anxiety. *Biological Psychology, 22,* 215–226.

Hermann, G., Beck, F. M., & Sheridan, J. F. (1995). Stress-induced glucocorticoid response modulates mononuclear cell trafficking during an experimental influenza viral infection. *Journal of Neuroimmunology, 56,* 179–186.

Higley, J. D., Suomi, S. J., & Linnoila, M. (1992). A longitudinal assessment of CSF monoamine metabolites and plasma cortisol concentrations in young rhesus monkeys. *Biological Psychiatry, 32,* 127–145.

Hines, E. A., Jr., & Brown, G. E. (1932). Standard stimulus for measuring vasomotor reactions: Its application in the study of hypertension. *Proceedings of the Staff Meetings of the Mayo Clinic, 7,* 332–335.

Hobbs, S. (1982). Central command during exercise: Parallel activation of the cardiovascular and motor systems by descending command signals. In O. A. Smith, R. A. Galosy, & S. M. Weiss (Eds.), *Circulation, neurobiology and behavior* (pp. 217–231). New York: Elsevier.

Hughes, J. W., Sherwood, A., Blumenthal, J. A., Suarez, E. C., & Hinderliter, A. L. (2003). Hostility, social support, and adrenergic receptor responsiveness among African-American and white men and women. *Psychosomatic Medicine, 65,* 582–587.

Huot, R. L., Thrivikraman, K. V., Meaney, M. J., & Plotsky, P. M. (2001). Development of adult ethanol preference and anxiety as a consequence of neonatal maternal separation in Long Evans rats and reversal with antidepressant treatment. *Psychopharmacology (Berlin), 158,* 366–373.

Jackson, A. S., Squires, W. G., Grimes, G., & Beard, E. F. (1983). Prediction of future resting hypertension from exercise blood pressure. *Journal of Cardiac Rehabilitation, 3,* 263–268.

Jansen, A. S., Nguyen, X. V., Karpitskiy, V., Mettenleiter, T. C., & Loewy, A. D. (1995). Central command neurons of the sympathetic nervous system: Basis of the fight-or-flight response. *Science, 270,* 644–646.

Jemmott, J., & Locke, S. (1984). Psychosocial factors, immunologic mediation, and human susceptibility to infectious diseases. *Psychological Bulletin, 95*, 78–108.

Jenkins, F. J., & Baum, A. (1995). Stress and reactivation of latent herpes simplex virus: A fusion of behavioral medicine and molecular biology. *Annals of Behavioral Medicine, 17*, 116–123.

Jiang, W., Babyak, M., Krantz, D. S., Waugh, R. A., Coleman, R. E., Hanson, M. M., et al. (1996). Mental stress–induced myocardial ischemia and cardiac events. *Journal of the American Medical Association, 275*, 1651–1656.

Kalin, N. H., Larson, C., Shelton, S. E., & Davidson, R. J. (1998). Asymmetric frontal brain activity, cortisol, and behavior associated with fearful temperament in rhesus monkeys. *Behavioral Neuroscience, 112*, 286–292.

Kamarck, T., & Jennings, J. R. (1991). Biobehavioral factors in sudden cardiac death. *Psychological Bulletin, 109*, 42–75.

Kamarck, T. W., & Lovallo, W. R. (2003). Cardiovascular reactivity to psychological challenge: Conceptual and measurement considerations. *Psychosomatic Medicine, 65*, 9–21.

Kandel, E. R., Schwartz, J. H., & Jessell, T. M. (2000). *Principles of neural science* (4th ed.). New York: McGraw-Hill.

Kaplan, J. R., Manuck, S. B., Clarkson, T. B., & Prichard, R. W. (1985). Animal models of behavioral influences on atherogenesis. In E. S. Katkin & S. B. Manuck (Eds.), *Advances in behavioral medicine* (pp. 115–164). Greenwich, CT: JAI.

Kark, J. D., Goldman, S., & Epstein, L. (1995). Iraqi missile attacks on Israel: The association of mortality with a life threatening stressor. *Journal of the American Medical Association, 273*, 1208–1210.

Kawachi, I., Colditz, G. A., Stampfer, M. J., Willett, W. C., Manson, J. E., Speizer, F. E., et al. (1995). Prospective study of shift work and risk of coronary heart disease in women. *Circulation, 92*, 3178–3182.

Keller, S. E., Shiflett, S. C., Schliefer, S. J., & Bartlett, J. A. (1994). Stress, immunity, and health. In R. Glaser & J. K. Kiecolt-Glaser (Eds.), *Handbook of human stress and immunity* (pp. 217–244). San Diego: Academic Press.

Kiecolt–Glaser, J. K., Malarkey, W. B., Cacioppo, J. T., & Glaser, R. (1994). Stressful personal relationships: Immune and endocrine function. In R. Glaser & J. K. Kiecolt-Glaser (Eds.), *Handbook of human stress and immunity* (pp. 321–339). San Diego: Academic Press.

Kiecolt-Glaser, J. K., Marucha, P. T., Malarkey, W. B., Mercado, A. M., & Glaser, R. (1995). Slowing of wound healing by psychological stress. *Lancet, 346*, 1194–1196.

Kiecolt-Glaser, J. K., McGuire, L., Robles, T. F., & Glaser, R. (2002). Psychoneuroimmunology and psychosomatic medicine: Back to the future. *Psychosomatic Medicine, 64*, 15–28.

Kirsch, I. (1990). *Changing expectations: A key to effective psychotherapy.* Pacific Grove, CA: Brooks/Cole.

Knardahl, S., & Hendley, E. D. (1990). Association between cardiovascular reactivity to stress and hypertension or behavior. *American Journal of Physiology, 259*, H248–H257.

Koepp, M. J., Gunn, R. N., Lawrence, A. D., Cunningham, V. J., Dagher, A., Jones, T., et al. (1998). Evidence for striatal dopamine release during a video game. *Nature, 393,* 266–268.

Kosslyn, S. M., & Koenig, O. (1995). *Wet mind: The new cognitive neuroscience* (2nd ed.). New York: Free Press.

Krantz, D. S., Quigley, J. F., & O'Callahan, M. (2001). Mental stress as a trigger of acute cardiac events: The role of laboratory studies. *Italian Heart Journal, 2,* 895–899.

Kreitler, S. (1999). Denial in cancer patients. *Cancer Investigations, 17,* 514–534.

Kuby, J. (1994). *Immunology* (2nd ed.). New York: W. H. Freeman.

Lampert, R., Joska, T., Burg, M. M., Batsford, W. P., McPherson, C. A., & Jain, D. (2002). Emotional and physical precipitants of ventricular arrhythmia. *Circulation, 106,* 1800–1805.

Laplante, P., Diorio, J., & Meaney, M. J. (2002). Serotonin regulates hippocampal glucocorticoid receptor expression via a 5-HT7 receptor. *Brain Research: Developmental Brain Research, 139,* 199–203.

Larson, M. R., Ader, R., & Moynihan, J. A. (2001). Heart rate, neuroendocrine, and immunological reactivity in response to an acute laboratory stressor. *Psychosomatic Medicine, 63,* 493–501.

Lazarus, R. S. (1991). *Emotion and adaptation.* New York: Oxford University Press.

Lazarus, R. S., & Folkman, S. (1984). *Stress, appraisal and coping.* New York: Springer.

LeDoux, J. E. (1993). Emotional memory systems in the brain. *Behavioral Brain Research, 58,* 69–79.

Leor, J., Poole, W. K., & Kloner, R. A. (1996). Sudden cardiac death triggered by an earthquake. *New England Journal of Medicine, 334,* 413–419.

Levenstein, S. (2000). The very model of a modern etiology: A biopsychosocial view of peptic ulcer. *Psychosomatic Medicine, 62,* 176–185.

Levine, S. (1957). Infantile experience and resistance to physiological stress. *Science, 126,* 405–406.

Levine, S. (2002). Regulation of the hypothalamic-pituitary-adrenal axis in the neonatal rat: The role of maternal behavior. *Neurotoxicity Research, 4,* 557–564.

Li, J., Precht, D. H., Mortensen, P. B., & Olsen, J. (2003). Mortality in parents after death of a child in Denmark: A nationwide follow-up study. *Lancet, 361,* 363–367.

Light, K. C., Dolan, C. A., Davis, M. R., & Sherwood, A. (1992). Cardiovascular responses to an active coping challenge as predictors of blood pressure patterns 10 to 15 years later. *Psychosomatic Medicine, 54,* 217–230.

Light, K. C., Girdler, S. S., Sherwood, A., Bragdon, E. E., Brownley, K. A., West, S. G., et al. (1999). High stress responsivity predicts later blood pressure only in combination with positive family history and high life stress. *Hypertension, 33,* 1458–1464.

Linden, W. (1991). What do arithmetic stress tests measure? Protocol variations and cardiovascular responses. *Psychophysiology, 28,* 91–102.

Linden, W., Gerin, W., & Davidson, K. (2003). Cardiovascular reactivity: Status quo and a research agenda for the new millennium. *Psychosomatic Medicine, 65,* 5–8.

Liu, D., Diorio, J., Tannenbaum, B., Caldji, C., Francis, D., Freedman, A., et al. (1997). Maternal care, hippocampal glucocorticoid receptors, and hypothalamic-pituitary-adrenal responses to stress. *Science, 277,* 1659–1662.

Lovallo, W. R., & al'Absi, M. (1998). Hemodynamics during rest and behavioral stress in normotensive men at high risk for hypertension. *Psychophysiology, 35,* 47–53.

Lovallo, W. R., al'Absi, M., & Pincomb, G. (2000). Caffeine raises blood pressure during extended mental stress in borderline hypertensive men. *International Journal of Behavioral Medicine, 7,* 183–188.

Lovallo, W. R., & Gerin, W. (2003). Psychophysiological reactivity: Mechanisms and pathways to cardiovascular disease. *Psychosomatic Medicine, 65,* 36–45.

Lovallo, W. R., Pincomb, G. A., Brackett, D. J., & Wilson, M. F. (1990). Heart rate reactivity as a predictor of neuroendocrine responses to aversive and appetitive challenges. *Psychosomatic Medicine, 52,* 17–26.

Lovallo, W. R., Pincomb, G. A., Sung, B. H., Everson, S. A., Passey, R. B., & Wilson, M. F. (1991). Hypertension risk and caffeine's effect on cardiovascular activity during mental stress in young men. *Health Psychology, 10,* 236–243.

Lovallo, W. R., Pincomb, G. A., & Wilson, M. F. (1986a). Heart rate reactivity and Type A behavior as modifiers of physiological response to active and passive coping. *Psychophysiology, 23,* 105–112.

Lovallo, W. R., Pincomb, G. A., & Wilson, M. F. (1986b). Predicting response to a reaction time task: Heart rate reactivity compared with Type A behavior. *Psychophysiology, 23,* 648–656.

Lovallo, W. R., & Wilson, M. F. (1992). The role of cardiovascular reactivity in hypertension risk. In J. R. Turner, A. Sherwood, & K. C. Light (Eds.), *Individual differences in cardiovascular response to stress* (pp. 165–186). New York: Plenum.

Lovallo, W. R., Wilson, M. F., Pincomb, G. A., Edwards, G. L., Tompkins, P., & Brackett, D. (1985). Activation patterns to aversive stimulation in man: Passive exposure versus effort to control. *Psychophysiology, 22,* 283–291.

Luger, A., Deuster, P. A., Kyle, S. B., Gallucci, W. T., Montgomery, L. C., Gold, P. W., et al. (1987). Acute hypothalamic-pituitary-adrenal responses to the stress of treadmill exercise. *New England Journal of Medicine, 316,* 1309–1315.

Lundberg, U., & Frankenhaeuser, M. (1980). Pituitary-adrenal and sympathetic-adrenal correlates of distress and effort. *Journal of Psychosomatic Research, 24,* 125–130.

Manuck, S. B., & Garland, F. N. (1980). Stability of individual differences in cardiovascular reactivity: A thirteen month follow-up. *Physiology & Behavior, 24,* 621–624.

Manuck, S. B., Kaplan, J. R., Adams, M. R., & Clarkson, T. B. (1989). Behaviorally elicited heart rate reactivity and atherosclerosis in female cynomolgus monkeys (*Macaca fascicularis*). *Psychosomatic Medicine, 51,* 306–318.

Marucha, P. T., Kiecolt-Glaser, J. K., & Favagehi, M. (1998). Mucosal wound healing is impaired by examination stress. *Psychosomatic Medicine, 60*, 362–365.

Mason, J. W. (1968). Organization of psychoendocrine mechanisms. *Psychosomatic Medicine, 30*, 565–808.

Mason, J. W. (1975a). An historical view of the stress field: Part I. *Journal of Human Stress, 1*(1), 6–12.

Mason, J. W. (1975b). An historical view of the stress field: Part II. *Journal of Human Stress, 1*(2), 22–35.

Matthews, K. A., Salomon, K., Brady, S. S., & Allen, M. T. (2003). Cardiovascular reactivity to stress predicts future blood pressure in adolescence. *Psychosomatic Medicine, 65*, 410–415.

McArdle, W. D., Foglia, G. F., & Patti, A. V. (1967). Telemetered cardiac response to selected running events. *Journal of Applied Physiology, 23*, 566–570.

McEwen, B. S., & Sapolsky, R. M. (1995). Stress and cognitive function. *Current Opinion in Neurobiology, 5*, 205–216.

McEwen, B. S., & Stellar, E. (1993). Stress and the individual: Mechanisms leading to disease. *Archives of Internal Medicine, 153*, 2093–2101.

McGaugh, J. L., & Roozendaal, B. (2002). Role of adrenal stress hormones in forming lasting memories in the brain. *Current Opinion in Neurobiology, 12*, 205–210.

McKinnon, W., Weisse, C. S., Reynolds, C. P., Bowles, C. A., & Baum, A. (1989). Chronic stress, leukocyte subpopulations, and humoral response to latent viruses. *Health Psychology, 8*, 389–402.

Meaney, M. J. (2001). Maternal care, gene expression, and the transmission of individual differences in stress reactivity across generations. *Annual Review of Neuroscience, 24*, 1161–1192.

Meaney, M. J., Aitken, D. H., Bodnoff, S. R., Iny, L. J., Tatarewicz, J. E., & Sapolsky, R. M. (1985). Early postnatal handling alters glucocorticoid receptor concentrations in selected brain regions. *Behavioral Neuroscience, 99*, 765–770.

Meaney, M. J., Brake, W., & Gratton, A. (2002). Environmental regulation of the development of mesolimbic dopamine systems: A neurobiological mechanism for vulnerability to drug abuse? *Psychoneuroendocrinology, 27*, 127–138.

Menkes, M. S., Matthews, K. A., Krantz, D. S., Lundberg, U., Mead, L. A., Quaqish, B., et al. (1989). Cardiovascular reactivity to the cold pressor test as a predictor of hypertension. *Hypertension, 14*, 524–530.

Merriam-Webster's collegiate dictionary (10th ed.). (1993). Springfield, MA: Merriam-Webster.

Miller, N. E. (1995). Clinical-experimental interactions in the development of neuroscience. *American Psychologist, 50*, 901–911.

Mills, P. J., Dimsdale, J. E., Nelesen, R. A., Jasiewicz, J., Ziegler, M. G., & Kennedy, B. (1994). Patterns of adrenergic receptors and adrenergic agonists underlying cardiovascular responses to a psychological challenge. *Psychosomatic Medicine, 56*, 70–76.

Mills, P. J., Dimsdale, J. E., Ziegler, M. G., Berry, C. C., & Bain, R. D. (1990). Beta-adrenergic receptors predict heart rate reactivity to a psychosocial stressor. *Psychosomatic Medicine, 52,* 621–623.

Milner, B., & Penfield, W. (1955). The effect of hippocampal lesions on recent memory. *Transactions of the American Neurological Association, 80,* 42–48.

Mittleman, M. A., Maclure, M., Sherwood, J. B., Mulry, R. P., Tofler, G. H., Jacobs, S. C., et al. (1995). Triggering of acute myocardial infarction onset by episodes of anger. *Circulation, 92,* 1720–1725.

Moncek, F., Kvetnansky, R., & Jezova, D. (2001). Differential responses to stress stimuli of Lewis and Fischer rats at the pituitary and adrenocortical level. *Endocrine Regulations, 35,* 35–41.

Monnot, M. (1999). Function of infant-directed speech. *Human Nature, 10,* 415–443.

Morell, V. (1995). Zeroing in on how hormones affect the immune system. *Science, 269,* 773–775.

Morentin, B., Suarez-Mier, M. P., & Aguilera, B. (2003). Sudden unexplained death among persons 1–35 years old. *Forensic Science International, 135,* 213–217.

Munck, A., Guyre, P. M., & Holbrook, N. J. (1984). Physiological functions of glucocorticoids in stress and their relation to pharmacological actions. *Endocrine Reviews, 5,* 25–44.

Neisser, U. (1967). *Cognitive psychology.* New York: Appleton-Century-Crofts.

Ottaway, C. A., & Husband, A. J. (1992). Central nervous system influences on lymphocyte migration. *Brain, Behavior, and Immunity, 69,* 97–116.

Padgett, D. A., Marucha, P. T., & Sheridan, J. F. (1998). Restraint stress slows cutaneous wound healing in mice. *Brain, Behavior, and Immunity, 12,* 64–73.

Petrusz, P., & Merchenthaler, I. (1992). The corticotropin-releasing factor system. In C. B. Nemeroff (Ed.), *Neuroendocrinology* (pp. 129–183). Boca Raton, FL: CRC Press.

Pincomb, G. A., Lovallo, W. R., McKey, B. S., Sung, B. H., Passey, R. B., Everson, S. A., et al. (1996). Acute blood pressure elevations with caffeine in men with borderline systemic hypertension. *American Journal of Cardiology, 77,* 270–274.

Plato. (1964). *The republic* (H. D. P. Lee, Trans.). Baltimore, MD: Penguin.

Plotsky, P. M., & Meaney, M. J. (1993). Early, postnatal experience alters hypothalamic corticotropin-releasing factor (CRF) mRNA, median eminence CRF content and stress-induced release in adult rats. *Brain Research: Molecular Brain Research, 18,* 195–200.

Premack, D. (2004). Psychology: Is language the key to human intelligence? *Science, 303,* 318–320.

Ramsay, D. S., & Woods, S. C. (2001). The use and usefulness of placebo controls. *Science, 294,* 785.

Rescorla, R. A. (1988). Pavlovian conditioning: It's not what you think it is. *American Psychology, 43,* 151–160.

Rojas, I. G., Padgett, D. A., Sheridan, J. F., & Marucha, P. T. (2002). Stress-induced susceptibility to bacterial infection during cutaneous wound healing. *Brain, Behavior, and Immunity, 16,* 74–84.

Roozendaal, B., Nguyen, B. T., Power, A. E., & McGaugh, J. L. (1999). Basolateral amygdala noradrenergic influence enables enhancement of memory consolidation induced by hippocampal glucocorticoid receptor activation. *Proceedings of the National Academy of Sciences USA, 96,* 11642–11647.

Roseboom, T. J., van der Meulen, J. H., Ravelli, A. C., Osmond, C., Barker, D. J., & Bleker, O. P. (2001). Effects of prenatal exposure to the Dutch famine on adult disease in later life: An overview. *Twin Research, 4,* 293–298.

Rozlog, L. A., Kiecolt-Glaser, J. K., Marucha, P. T., Sheridan, J. F., & Glaser, R. (1999). Stress and immunity: Implications for viral disease and wound healing. *Journal of Periodontology, 70,* 786–792.

Rushmer, R. M. (1989). Structure and function of the cardiovascular system. In N. Schneiderman, P. Kaufmann, & S. Weiss (Eds.), *Handbook of research methods in cardiovascular behavioral medicine* (pp. 5–22). New York: Plenum.

Ryle, G. (1949). *The concept of mind.* London: Hutchinson.

Saini, V., & Verrier, R. L. (1989). The experimental study of behaviorally induced arrhythmias. In N. Schneiderman, P. Kaufmann, & S. Weiss (Eds.), *Handbook of research methods in cardiovascular behavioral medicine* (pp. 51–68). New York: Plenum.

Sapolsky, R. M. (1996). Why stress is bad for your brain. *Science, 273,* 749–750.

Sausen, K. P., Lovallo, W. R., Pincomb, G. A., & Wilson, M. F. (1992). Cardiovascular responses to occupational stress in medical students: A paradigm for ambulatory monitoring studies. *Health Psychology, 11,* 55–60.

Scheinman, R. I., Cogswell, P. C., Lofquist, A. K., & Baldwin, A. S. (1995). Role of transcriptional activation of IκBα in mediation of immunosuppression by glucocorticoids. *Science, 270,* 283–286.

Schommer, N. C., Hellhammer, D. H., & Kirschbaum, C. (2003). Dissociation between reactivity of the hypothalamus-pituitary-adrenal axis and the sympathetic-adrenal-medullary system to repeated psychosocial stress. *Psychosomatic Medicine, 65,* 450–460.

Schulkin, J., Gold, P. W., & McEwen, B. S. (1998). Induction of corticotropin-releasing hormone gene expression by glucocorticoids: Implication for understanding the states of fear and anxiety and allostatic load. *Psychoneuroendocrinology, 23,* 219–243.

Schulkin, J., McEwen, B. S., & Gold, P. W. (1994). Allostasis, amygdala and anticipatory angst. *Neuroscience and Behavioral Reviews, 18,* 385–396.

Schwartz, A. R., Gerin, W., Davidson, K. W., Pickering, T. G., Brosschot, J. F., Thayer, J. F., et al. (2003). Toward a causal model of cardiovascular responses to stress and the development of cardiovascular disease. *Psychosomatic Medicine, 65,* 22–35.

Schwartz, G. (1979). The brain as a health care system. In G. C. Stone, F. Cohen, & N. E. Adler (Eds.), *Health psychology: A handbook* (pp. 549–571). San Francisco: Jossey-Bass.

Schwartz, J. M., Stoessel, P. W., Baxter, L. R., Jr., Martin, K. M., & Phelps, M. E. (1996). Systematic changes in cerebral glucose metabolic rate after successful behavior modification treatment of obsessive-compulsive disorder. *Archives of General Psychiatry, 53,* 109–113.

Scoville, W. B., & Milner, B. (2000). Loss of recent memory after bilateral hippocampal lesions. 1957. *Journal of Neuropsychiatry Clinics of Neurosciences, 12,* 103–113.

Seligman, M. E. P., Maier, S., & Solomon, R.L. (1971). Unpredictable and uncontrollable aversive events. In F. R. Brush (Ed.), *Aversive conditioning and learning* (pp. 347–400). New York: Academic Press.

Selye, H. (1936). Thymus and adrenals in the response of the organism to injuries and intoxications. *British Journal of Experimental Pathology, 17,* 234–248.

Selye, H. (1956). *The stress of life.* New York: McGraw-Hill.

Sgoutas-Emch, S. A., Cacioppo, J. T., Uchino, B. N., Malarkey, W., Pearl, D., Kiecolt-Glaser, J. K., et al. (1994). The effects of an acute psychological stressor on cardiovascular, endocrine, and cellular immune response: A prospective study of individuals high and low in heart rate reactivity. *Psychophysiology, 31,* 264–271.

Shepard, J. D., Barron, K. W., & Myers, D. A. (2000). Corticosterone delivery to the amygdala increases corticotropin-releasing factor mRNA in the central amygdaloid nucleus and anxiety-like behavior. *Brain Research, 861,* 288–295.

Shepard, J. D., Barron, K. W., & Myers, D. A. (2003). Stereotaxic localization of corticosterone to the amygdala enhances hypothalamo-pituitary-adrenal responses to behavioral stress. *Brain Research, 963,* 203–213.

Sheridan, J. F., & Dobbs, C. M. (1994). Stress, viral pathogenesis, and immunity. In R. Glaser & J. Kiecolt-Glaser (Eds.), *Handbook of human stress and immunity* (pp. 101–123). San Diego: Academic Press.

Sherwood, A., Girdler, S. S., Bragdon, E. E., West, S. G., Brownley, K. A., Hinderliter, A. L., et al. (1997). Ten-year stability of cardiovascular responses to laboratory stressors. *Psychophysiology, 34,* 185–191.

Sherwood, A., & Turner, J. R. (1992). A conceptual and methodological overview of cardiovascular reactivity research. In J. R. Turner, A. Sherwood, & K. C. Light (Eds.), *Individual differences in cardiovascular response to stress* (pp. 3–32). New York: Plenum.

Siegler, I. C., Costa, P. T., Brummett, B. H., Helms, M. J., Barefoot, J. C., Williams, R. B., et al. (2003). Patterns of change in hostility from college to midlife in the UNC Alumni Heart Study predict high-risk status. *Psychosomatic Medicine, 65,* 738–745.

Sloan, R. P., Bagiella, E., Shapiro, P. A., Kuhl, J. P., Chernikhova, D., Berg, J., et al. (2001). Hostility, gender, and cardiac autonomic control. *Psychosomatic Medicine, 63,* 434–440.

Smith, E. E., Guyton, A. C., Manning, R. D., & White, R. J. (1976). Integrated mechanisms of cardiovascular response and control during exercise in the normal human. *Progress in Cardiovascular Disease, 28,* 421–443.

Smith, O. A., Astley, C. A., Spelman, F. A., Golanov, E. V., Chalyan, V. G., Bowden, D. M., et al. (1993). Integrating behavior and cardiovascular responses: Posture and locomotion. I. Static analysis. *American Journal of Physiology, 265,* R1458–R1468.

Smith, O. A., DeVito, J. L., & Astley, C. A. (1982). Cardiovascular control centers in the brain: One more look. In O. A. Smith, R. A. Galosy, & S. M. Weiss (Eds.), *Circulation, neurobiology and behavior* (pp. 233–246). New York, NY: Elsevier.

Solomon, G. F., & Benton, D. (1994). Psychoneuroimmunologic aspects of aging. In R. Glaser & J. Kiecolt-Glaser (Eds.), *Handbook of human stress and immunity* (pp. 341–363). San Diego: Academic Press.

Soufer, R., Bremner, J. D., Arrighi, J. A., Cohen, I., Zaret, B. L., Burg, M. M., et al. (1998). Cerebral cortical hyperactivation in response to mental stress in patients with coronary artery disease. *Proceedings of the National Academy of Sciences USA, 95,* 6454–6459.

Stanton, M. E., Gutierrez, Y. R., & Levine, S. (1988). Maternal deprivation potentiates pituitary-adrenal stress responses in infant rats. *Behavioral Neuroscience, 102,* 692–700.

Sterling, P., & Eyer, J. (1988). Allostasis: A new paradigm to explain arousal pathology. In S. Fisher & J. Reason (Eds.), *Handbook of life stress, cognition, and health* (pp. 629–649). New York: John Wiley.

Sternberg, E. M., Hill, J. M., Chrousos, G. P., Kamilaris, T., Listwak, S. J., Gold, P. W., et al. (1989). Inflammatory mediator-induced hypothalamic-pituitary-adrenal axis activation is defective in streptococcal cell wall arthritis susceptible Lewis rats. *Proceedings of the National Academy of Sciences USA, 86,* 2374–2378.

Sternberg, E. M., Wilder, R. L., Chrousos, G. P., & Gold, P. W. (1991). Stress responses and the pathogenesis of arthritis. In J. A. McCubbin, P. G. Kaufmann, & C. B. Nemeroff (Eds.), *Stress, neuropeptides, and systemic disease* (pp. 287–300). New York: Academic Press.

Stone, A. A., Neale, J. M., Cox, D. S., Napoli, A., Valdimarsdottir, H., & Kennedy-Moore, E. (1994). Daily events are associated with a secretory immune response to an oral antigen in men. *Health Psychology, 13,* 440–446.

Suarez, E. C. (2003). Joint effect of hostility and severity of depressive symptoms on plasma interleukin-6 concentration. *Psychosomatic Medicine, 65,* 523–527.

Suarez, E. C., Kuhn, C. M., Schanberg, S. M., Williams, R. B., Jr., & Zimmermann, E. A. (1998). Neuroendocrine, cardiovascular, and emotional responses of hostile men: The role of interpersonal challenge. *Psychosomatic Medicine, 60,* 78–88.

Suarez, E. C., & Williams, R. B. (1989). Situational determinants of cardiovascular and emotional reactivity in high and low hostile men. *Psychosomatic Medicine, 51,* 404–418.

Sung, B. H., Lovallo, W. R., Whitsett, T., & Wilson, M. F. (1995). Caffeine elevates blood pressure response to exercise in mild-hypertensive men. *American Journal of Hypertension, 8,* 1184–1188.

Sung, B. H., Wilson, M. F., Robinson, C., Thadani, U., & Lovallo, W. R. (1988). Mechanisms of myocardial ischemia induced by epinephrine: Comparison with exercise-induced ischemia. *Psychosomatic Medicine, 50,* 381–393.

Timio, M., Verdecchia, P., Venanzi, S., Gentili, S., Ronconi, M., Francucci, B., et al. (1988). Age and blood pressure changes: A 20-year follow-up study in nuns in a secluded order. *Hypertension, 12,* 457–461.

Tomarken, A. J., Davidson, R. J., Wheeler, R. E., & Doss, R. C. (1992). Individual differences in anterior brain asymmetry and fundamental dimensions of emotion. *Journal of Personality and Social Psychology, 62,* 676–687.

Toulmin, S. (1967). Neuroscience and human understanding. In G. C. Quarton, T. Melnechuk, & F. O. Schmitt (Eds.), *The neurosciences: A study program* (pp. 822–832). New York: Rockefeller University Press.

Treiber, F. A., Kamarck, T., Schneiderman, N., Sheffield, D., Kapuku, G., & Taylor, T. (2003). Cardiovascular reactivity and development of preclinical and clinical disease states. *Psychosomatic Medicine, 65,* 46–62.

Turner, J. R., & Carroll, D. (1985). Heart rate and oxygen consumption during mental arithmetic, a video game, and graded exercise: Further evidence of metabolically exaggerated cardiac adjustments? *Psychophysiology, 22,* 261–267.

Uchino, B. N., Cacioppo, R. T., Malarkey, W., & Glaser, R. (1995). Individual differences in cardiac sympathetic control predict endocrine and immune responses to acute psychological stress. *Journal of Personality and Social Psychology, 69,* 736–743.

Ungerleider, L. G. (1995). Functional brain imaging studies of cortical mechanisms for memory. *Science, 270,* 769–775.

van Oers, H. J., de Kloet, E. R., & Levine, S. (1998). Early vs. late maternal deprivation differentially alters the endocrine and hypothalamic responses to stress. *Brain Research: Developmental Brain Research, 111,* 245–252.

van Oers, H. J., de Kloet, E. R., Whelan, T., & Levine, S. (1998). Maternal deprivation effect on the infant's neural stress markers is reversed by tactile stimulation and feeding but not by suppressing corticosterone. *Journal of Neuroscience, 18,* 10171–10179.

Vazquez, D. M., Lopez, J. F., Van Hoers, H., Watson, S. J., & Levine, S. (1999). Maternal deprivation regulates serotonin 1A and 2A receptors in the infant rat. *Brain Research, 855,* 76–82.

Vitaliano, P. P., Zhang, J., & Scanlon, J. (2003). Is caregiving hazardous to one's physical health? A meta-analysis. *Psychological Bulletin, 129,* 946–972.

Watson, M., Greer, S., Blake, S., & Shrapnell, K. (1984). Reaction to a diagnosis of breast cancer: Relationship between denial, delay and rates of psychological morbidity. *Cancer, 53,* 2008–2012.

Weaver, I. C., Grant, R. J., & Meaney, M. J. (2002). Maternal behavior regulates long-term hippocampal expression of BAX and apoptosis in the offspring. *Journal of Neurochemistry, 82,* 998–1002.

Weaver, S. A., Aherne, F. X., Meaney, M. J., Schaefer, A. L., & Dixon, W. T. (2000). Neonatal handling permanently alters hypothalamic-pituitary-adrenal axis function, behaviour, and body weight in boars. *Journal of Endocrinology, 164,* 349–359.

Webster's ninth new collegiate dictionary. (1988). Springfield, MA: Merriam-Webster.

Weiner, H. (1991a). From simplicity to complexity (1950–1990): The case of peptic ulceration: I. Human studies. *Psychosomatic Medicine, 53,* 467–490.

Weiner, H. (1991b). From simplicity to complexity (1950–1990): The case of peptic ulceration: II. Animal studies. *Psychosomatic Medicine, 53,* 491–516.

Weiner, H. (1992). *Perturbing the organism: The biology of stressful experience.* Chicago: University of Chicago Press.

Weiss, J. M. (1970). Somatic effects of predictable and unpredictable shock. *Psychosomatic Medicine, 32,* 397–408.

Weiss, J. M. (1971a). Effects of coping behavior in different warning-signal conditions on stress pathology in rats. *Journal of Comparative and Physiological Psychology, 77,* 1–13.

Weiss, J. M. (1971b). Effects of coping behavior with and without a feedback signal on stress pathology in rats. *Journal of Comparative and Physiological Psychology, 77,* 22–30.

Weiss, J. M. (1980). Part V: Explaining behavioral depression following uncontrollable stressful events. *Behavioral Research and Therapy, 18,* 485–504.

Weiss, J. M. (1991). Stress-induced depression: Critical neurochemical and electrophysiological changes. In I. J. Madden (Ed.), *Neurobiology of learning, emotion and affect* (pp. 123–154). New York: Raven.

Weiss, J. M., Goodman, P. A., Losito, B. G., Corrigan, S., Charry, J. M., & Bailey, W. H. (1981). Behavioral depression produced by an uncontrollable stressor: Relationship to norepinephrine, dopamine, and serotonin levels in various regions of rat brain. *Brain Research Reviews, 3,* 167–205.

Weiss, J. M., Simson, P. G., Ambrose, M. J., Webster, A., & Hoffman, L. J. (1985). Neurochemical basis of behavioral depression. In E. S. Katkin & S. B. Manuck (Eds.), *Advances in behavioral medicine* (Vol. 1, pp. 233–276). Greenwich, CT: JAI.

Weiss, J. M., & Sundar, S. (1992). Effects of stress on cellular immune responses in animals. In A. Tasman & M. Riba (Eds.), *Review of psychiatry* (Vol. 11, pp. 145–168). Washington, DC: American Psychiatric Press.

Williams, R. B. (1994). Neurobiology, cellular and molecular biology, and psychosomatic medicine. *Psychosomatic Medicine, 56,* 308–315.

Williams, R. B., Jr., Lane, J. D., Kuhn, C. M., Melosh, W., White, A. D., & Schanberg, S. M. (1982). Type A behavior and elevated physiological and neuroendocrine responses to cognitive tasks. *Science, 218,* 483–485.

Wilson, M. F., Sung, B. H., Pincomb, G. A., & Lovallo, W. R. (1990). Exaggerated pressure response to exercise in men at risk for systemic hypertension. *American Journal of Cardiology, 66,* 731–736.

Wilson, N. V., & Meyer, B. M. (1981). Early prediction of hypertension using exercise blood pressure. *Preventive Medicine, 10,* 62–68.

Yang, E. V., & Glaser, R. (2002). Stress-associated immunomodulation and its implications for responses to vaccination. *Expert Review of Vaccines, 1,* 453–459.

Zhang, L. X., Levine, S., Dent, G., Zhan, Y., Xing, G., Okimoto, D., et al. (2002). Maternal deprivation increases cell death in the infant rat brain. *Brain Research: Developmental Brain Research, 133,* 1–11.

Author Index

Subject Index

About the Author

William R. Lovallo, Ph.D., is Professor of Psychiatry and Behavioral Sciences at the University of Oklahoma Health Sciences Center and Director of the Behavioral Sciences Laboratories at the VA Medical Center, Oklahoma City. His research has been supported by the United States Department of Veterans Affairs, the National Institutes of Health, and the John D. and Catherine T. MacArthur Foundation. He has devoted his career to the study of stress mechanisms and risk for cardiovascular disease. In 2000 he finished six years as Associate Director of the MacArthur Foundation's Research Network on Mind-Body Interactions in Chicago, where he also served as Professor of Psychiatry and Behavioral Sciences and Professor of Psychology at Rush-Presbyterian-St. Luke's Medical Center. He has served on editorial boards of the *International Journal of Psychophysiology, Psychosomatic Medicine, International Journal of Behavioral Medicine,* and *Annals of Behavioral Medicine.*